# To Improve Health and Health Care

## Volume XVI

Stephen L. Isaacs and
David C. Colby, Editors
Foreword by Risa Lavizzo-Mourey

# —⁓—To Improve Health and Health Care

## Volume XVI

The Robert Wood Johnson
Foundation Anthology

# JB JOSSEY-BASS™
A Wiley Brand

Cover design by Wiley
Cover image : © Dave Cutler Studios

Published by Jossey-Bass
A Wiley Brand
One Montgomery Street, Suite 1200, San Francisco, CA 94104-4594-www.josseybass.com

Jossey-Bass books and products are available through most bookstores. To contact Jossey-Bass directly call our Customer Care Department within the U.S. at 800-956-7739, outside the U.S. at 317-572-3986, or fax 317-572-4002.

Wiley publishes in a variety of print and electronic formats and by print-on-demand. Some material included with standard print versions of this book may not be included in e-books or in print-on-demand. If this book refers to media such as a CD or DVD that is not included in the version you purchased, you may download this material at http://booksupport.wiley.com. For more information about Wiley products, visit www.wiley.com.

ISSN: 1547-3570
ISBN: 978-111-9-00078-5

Printed in the United States of America
FIRST EDITION
PB Printing 10 9 8 7 6 5 4 3 2 1

# —ᴡᴡ—Contents

# —⚊—Foreword: Crafting a New Vision for the Robert Wood Johnson Foundation

*Risa Lavizzo-Mourey*

The theme of this year's *Anthology* is discovery—discovery of new ideas and innovations; discovery of approaches to solve seemingly intractable social problems; discovery of ways to transform a routine city hotline into one serving a new group of needy individuals.

The volume begins with a chapter that explains how the Foundation finds ideas. That is followed by three chapters on the pioneer portfolio. One describes the pioneer team's approach to seeking out innovators, and the other two highlight new ways to solve problems that the pioneer team discovered and the Foundation funded—sharing physicians' notes with patients through the Open Notes program, and using video games to promote health.

The next five chapters examine how the Foundation has been addressing one of the nation's most important health issues, the epidemic of childhood obesity. These chapters present the Foundation's approach to reducing childhood obesity, look at the policy research generated by Foundation grantees, describe Foundation-funded efforts to enhance the built environment, and examine programs to improve nutrition in the nation's schools (the Healthy Schools program) and to combat childhood obesity at the community level (the Healthy Kids, Healthy Communities program).

The volume concludes with a chapter on how committed individuals found a way to use Los Angeles County's 211 social services hotline to identify children with developmental disabilities and refer them to the services they need.

A book about discovery resonated with me, for, beginning in mid-2012, the Foundation went through its own process of discovery as we crafted a strategic plan whose centerpiece was an entirely new vision. We were looking to build upon the Foundation's work over its forty-year history to find bold ways to help make the United States a healthier nation. The process took more than a year, involved the entire staff, and was overseen by the Board of Trustees.[1] From the very beginning, the Board instructed us to cast a wide net and avoid simply making incremental changes that would look to the past but not the future. It admonished us not to repeat the mistakes of the eighteenth-century British, who wasted their time building speedier sailing ships just as steam-powered ships were rendering them obsolete.

Our discovery process began with a concerted effort to learn everything we could about what health and health care were likely to look like in the future. We sought the counsel of experts. We compiled, read, and discussed the most thoughtful analyses of where health and health care were heading. And we examined the issues in staff meetings and retreats, including an all-staff "learning session," in which participants were asked to consider how health and health care were likely to change over the next twenty years, what the Foundation's blind spots were, and how the Foundation could improve its work.

To provide a context for the learning session, the Foundation commissioned the Institute for Alternative Futures to explore four scenarios for health and health care between 2013 and 2032. The first was slow reform accompanied by improved health (largely through prevention); the second was a worsening of the current system, with a consequent deterioration of health; the third was using Big Data to generate major health gains; and the fourth was creation of a culture of health.

As a result of these various efforts, we were able to identify trends that should inform the Foundation's work in the future, among them:

- The population will become simultaneously older and more diverse, with the highest concentration of diversity among the youngest segments.

- Tension will increase between investing in an increasingly aging population and investing in younger people.

- Education and income disparities will increase.

- Nonmedical determinants of health, such as education, income, employment, and environmental factors, will become increasingly associated with health outcomes.

- Overall spending on health care will continue to pose a significant challenge for individuals and society.

- Media and communication tools will continue to change how we collect, aggregate, and share health and health care information.

- Breakthroughs in fields such as genomics and neuroscience, along with powerful new data analysis tools, will continue to inform our knowledge about what influences health, strategies to prevent and treat disease, and the root causes of poor health.

- Financial incentives will shift toward rewarding effective treatment and improved health outcomes.

- The locus of care will shift from the doctor's office to the community.

The next step in our process of discovery was trying to understand how the Foundation could have more influence in bringing about the kinds of changes that would lead to a healthier America. For answers to this, we reached beyond health and health care and sought the guidance of experts in other fields. We asked five luminaries to prepare analyses based on their expertise and to lead a discussion at a second all-staff learning session. The experts were Sinan Aral, an MIT professor and leading expert on social media and networks; Dan Ariely, a highly regarded behavioral economist and author of *Predictably Irrational*; Sara Horowitz, the creator of the Freelancers Union and winner of a MacArthur Foundation Genius Award; Michelle McMurry-Heath, a physician and biochemist who is currently a high-ranking official at the US Food and Drug Administration; and Dan Wagner, a data analysis expert widely credited for the voter microtargeting that helped swing the 2012 presidential election.

Among the insights to emerge were the following:

- Human irrationality is a powerful force.

- Old beliefs often persist in the face of overwhelming evidence.

- The tiniest units of human behavior can be micro-targeted.

- Being influential in the age of networks requires mastering an emerging body of science focused on things like diffusion models and causality mapping.

- Technology and data are not the answer. As important as these are, change happens when people are moved.

- Environments and processes that are engineered to make it easier to do the right thing can have great impact on healthy decision making.

- In a networked world of decentralized power and suspicion of experts—one where innovation often comes from crosscutting teams working together toward a goal—successful leaders will need new skills and sensibilities.

- Tomorrow's America will be both better connected and more siloed along the lines of affinity groups, sectors, disciplines, industries, geographies, and the like. That apparent tension must be reconciled.

Proceeding along a parallel track, the Foundation's teams were reviewing their own successes and failures and were consulting their grantees, colleagues, and consultants for ideas about how their work, and that of the Foundation, could be improved. The teams presented their ideas and plans to the senior staff, which guided the strategic planning process. In addition, recognizing that its work did not exist in a vacuum, the Foundation commissioned analyses of what other foundations in health and related fields were doing.

This process of discovery culminated in the decision to adopt a new vision—one that would commit the Foundation to advancing "a culture of health." This new vision is not simply tinkering; it is new and aspirational, and gives the Foundation the opportunity to stimulate a nationwide conversation about what it means to be healthy and how the *nation* can become healthier. This vision reaches the very essence of society—its values.

In a way, the new vision completes a transition. Between 1972 and 1990, the Foundation focused almost exclusively on improving health care; from 1991 through 2013, it was devoted to improving both health care and health. With its new vision, the Foundation can concentrate on the nation's health. This does not signify that we are abandoning or minimizing our commitment to improving access to affordable and high-quality health care. Rather, we view health care as one important contributor to health, along with behavior, genetics, and the socioeconomic environment in which people live. We are aware of the many challenges the new vision will entail, but we are prepared to meet them. And we are in it for the long haul.

## Note

1. Monitor/Deloitte and Health Policy Associates provided guidance during the strategic planning process.

# —⌇⌇—Acknowledgments

We are grateful to all those whose efforts made this volume of *To Improve Health and Health Care XVI: The Robert Wood Johnson Foundation Anthology* possible. Within the Foundation itself, Risa Lavizzo-Mourey has given the *Anthology* her full support at all times; Fred Mann has provided wise counsel; Mimi Turi, Megha Sanghavi, Marianne Brandmaier, and Carol Owle handled financial management adeptly; Hope Woodhead supervised the design and distribution of the book, aided by Joan Barlow; Mayra Saenz also helped with the book's distribution; Patti Higgins did internal fact checking and copy editing, giving us the assurance that dates and monetary amounts are accurate; Rose Littman, Tina Hines, and Joan McKay were invaluable in arranging meetings between the San Francisco–based editor and the staff at the Robert Wood Johnson Foundation; Carole Harris served as a link between the Princeton/Washington-based editor and the San Francisco-based editor; Mary Beth Kren was invaluable in locating hard-to-find documents and reports; Andrew Harrison provided materials from the Foundation's archives, including the oral history; Deb Malloy, who has been of immense help in a variety of ways since the *Anthology* series began, assisted this year in reviewing chapters prior to their being posted on the Foundation's Web site; and Alexa Juarez provided research assistance in gathering materials for authors.

We wish to thank those who read chapters in draft form and who offered helpful comments on all or some of them—Risa

Lavizzo-Mourey, Fred Mann, Dwayne Proctor, Paul Tarini, and Brian Quinn.

Special thanks are due to four Foundation staff members. Molly McKaughan, who has collaborated with the *Anthology* editors for many years, suggested topics, recommended authors, and cast a keen editorial eye on every chapter. Amy Woodrum, an extraordinarily talented research assistant, carried out the task of gathering information for the authors with alacrity and good cheer and, in addition, conducted research, did fact checking, and helped with the editing. She was a partner in all aspects of this publication. Penny Bolla was the model of efficiency and commitment in seeing that chapters were posted to the Web in a timely and accurate fashion. Sherry DeMarchi did what can only be termed an amazing job handling the distribution of the book and in bringing the mailing list up to date.

Beyond the Foundation's staff, we are indebted to Susan Dentzer and Jim Knickman for serving as the outside reviewers for the *Anthology*. Their analysis of the draft chapters strengthened the volume immeasurably. Jim Morgan, our copyeditor, once again added grace to the prose in every chapter. Carolyn Shea continues to be without peer as a fact checker. Ilan Isaacs proofread the galleys and caught errors that had escaped other readers.

At Jossey-Bass, we thank Seth Schwartz, Justin Frahm, Melinda Noack, and Donna Jane Askay.

Finally, we are saddened by the death of Andy Pasternack in 2013. Andy, who as the health series editor at Jossey-Bass, was a partner in the *Anthology* series from its birth. He was a tireless supporter, an able problem-solver, and, most important, an extraordinarily decent human being.

SLI/DCC

# To Improve Health and Health Care

## Volume XVI

# Section One
# The Pioneer Portfolio

# Where Do Ideas Come From? The Robert Wood Johnson Foundation Experience

*David C. Colby, Stephen L. Isaacs, and Amy Woodrum*

Terry Keenan was a slight man whose courtly manner and gentle nature belied his background as a prizefighter and a Navy aviator. Considered *the* legendary Robert Wood Johnson Foundation grantmaker, Keenan was renowned for tramping through the Alaskan tundra and walking inner-city ghettoes in the dead of night in search of creative people and innovative ideas. He believed that philanthropy was the venture capital arm of society and that, as one of its representatives, he was obligated to unearth new and exciting approaches and to bring them to the attention of the Foundation.

Keenan would probably be considered an anachronism today, a charming relic of a time rendered obsolete by technology and the Internet. Nowadays, the search for ideas is less the province of hearty individuals personally interviewing health aides in Alaska or gang leaders in Chicago and more the province of people exchanging ideas on their computers or sitting around conference tables in foundation offices or hotel meeting rooms.

Much of the change has been driven by technology and the sheer quantity of information within easy reach. As Jack Welch, the former chairman of General Electric, once said, "The Internet is the single most important event in the U.S. economy since the Industrial Revolution."[1] The Internet makes it possible to find ideas from just about anywhere without lifting a finger (except to type on a keyboard) and vaults networking into a privileged position. In his book *Where Good Ideas Come From*, Steven Johnson finds that "every important innovation is fundamentally a network affair."[2] Ideas, he writes, begin as "slow hunches" and become fully formed through networks, largely technological ones that connect those hunches with those of others working in related areas.

The technological revolution has also upended the importance of expertise, replacing it with "crowdsourcing" and similar ways of generating ideas from a wide variety of people. *New Yorker* writer James Surowiecki argues that the best ideas come from the consensus of a great many people. "Heretical or not," he writes in *The Wisdom of Crowds,* "it's the truth; the value of expertise is, in many contexts, overrated . . . . If you can assemble a diverse group of people who possess varying degrees of knowledge and insight, you're better off entrusting it with major decisions than leaving it in the hands of one or two people."[3]

The pioneer portfolio, which is one of the two focal areas of this volume of *The Robert Wood Johnson Foundation Anthology*, has employed many of the latest approaches and technologies to seek out fresh ideas and new faces. It employs crowdsourcing, for example, and actively solicits ideas from outsiders through such vehicles as "Pitch Day," where entrepreneurs pitch Foundation officials on the "new new thing" in health.

As we thought about Tony Proscio's chapter on the pioneer portfolio,[4] it made us wonder how the Foundation got its ideas for programs in the past and just how significant the change from past to present (and future) really are. How, in short, has and does the Foundation find fresh program ideas and stay ahead of the curve?

## —∿— Finding Ideas 1: At the Beginning

When the Foundation was established in 1972, there was little time to develop programs because it faced a requirement of spending about $60 million quickly and doing it in a responsible manner. Foundation staff members could not devote a great deal of time to developing ideas and did not have the leisure to implement pilot projects to test ideas. Instead, they turned to ideas that could be funded rapidly—and were noncontroversial and safe to boot. Early grants could not entail reputational risks and, at their best, should enhance the Foundation's reputation.

In those early days, the Foundation relied on the expertise of its staff to find ideas and people. That staff, however, was extremely well connected, and it sought the counsel of former colleagues and other knowledgeable people in the health care field. One of the first things David Rogers, the Foundation's first president, did was to embark on a "listening tour," getting advice on directions the Foundation might take from health care experts and executives of other foundations.

Funding familiar activities and people and taking already existing programs from other foundations were two approaches that the Foundation used at the time. "We decided there were some safe areas that would not require a lot of supervision," said Rogers in a 1991 interview for the Foundation's oral history, looking back on the early days. Since Rogers was a physician and had been dean of a medical school prior to coming to the Robert Wood Johnson Foundation, providing scholarships to medical students was a familiar way to make the required payout. The first grant from the new foundation was to the Association of American Medical Colleges to manage a medical school scholarship program for women, minorities, and people from rural areas.

It was later expanded to include dental students. While the evaluation of the medical and dental student scholarship program questioned whether scholarships were the best way to target the money, it clearly was a safe bet for the new foundation. Once the Foundation developed a pipeline of projects, the funding of scholarships became far more targeted and took up a smaller piece of the pie.

In 1973, the Foundation started what was later internally referred to as "the Great Men" awards. These constituted grants to leading researchers who were well known to the Foundation's staff: Victor Fuchs, a health economist; David Mechanic, a medical sociologist; Eli Ginzberg, another health economist; and William Schwartz, a physician researcher. There was no request for proposals. These grant applications had neither methodological discussions nor tight foci; they were meant to support these scholars in the broad areas of their work.

Supporting these highly successful scholars was a safe bet that enhanced the reputation of the new foundation by its association with respected researchers. Allowing them freedom to pursue interesting topics was meant to encourage creativity. In many ways, it was a forerunner of pioneer portfolio's approach.

Another early mechanism the Foundation used to meet the payout requirement was to take over a program that had been started by others. This is how the Foundation came to sponsor the Clinical Scholars Program, which the Carnegie Corporation of New York and the Commonwealth Fund had established a few years previously. When David Rogers hired Margaret Mahoney away from Carnegie, he promised that she could bring the Clinical Scholars Program with her. About the same time, the Foundation hired Keenan from the Commonwealth Fund, the other funder of the Clinical Scholars Program. Leighton Cluff, the second president of the Foundation, explained in an interview for the Foundation's oral history in 1991, "Adoption of the Clinical Scholars Program was largely because the Foundation at that time was looking for programs to launch. It was just getting started, it had money to give away, and here was an already-established program that looked like it might have merit."

## —∿— Finding Ideas 2: The Traditional Robert Wood Johnson Foundation Approach

Once the Foundation had become better established, it developed a grantmaking model that has served it throughout most of its existence. The model relies on the knowledge and judgment of the Foundation's senior staff and program officers to determine over-all priorities and to develop programs to address the problems in the priority areas. The staff almost always consults knowledgeable people in the field—either formally or informally—as it does its research and makes these determinations.

Generally speaking, the Board of Trustees, which makes the final decisions, sets out broad outlines for programmatic approaches based on the president's recommendations (which are, of course, informed by the staff). In the 1990s, for example, when Steven Schroeder assumed the Foundation's presidency, the Board decided to concentrate on three priorities: reducing the harm caused by substance abuse; increasing access to health care; and improving the way services are provided to people with chronic health conditions. In 2003, when Risa Lavizzo-Mourey became the president and chief executive officer, the Board approved an Impact Framework that established new program priorities that guided the Foundation until 2014.

Once the Board sets the general direction, the Foundation staff, working in teams and seeking the advice of outside experts, hones the priorities into manageable program areas. To implement the programs, the Foundation usually issues calls for proposals that define what the Foundation wants to achieve and how it expects to get the results it hopes for. This often leads to the Foundation establishing a national program office, which oversees implemen-tation and recommends grants to carry out the program at specific sites. The Foundation names a national advisory committee to advise the national program office. Thus, in both seeking ideas and implementing programs, although the Foundation makes the final decisions, those decisions are arrived at in a collaborative manner within the Foundation after seeking guidance from outside experts.

Within this overall framework, the Foundation has taken a variety of approaches in seeking ideas for priorities and programs. Here are some examples of how the traditional approach has worked in practice.

### Copying or Expanding a Model

Over the Foundation's history, searching for programs that are successfully addressing a problem has been a dominant source of ideas for programs. Usually, these are programs already under way somewhere at the city or state level. Through this mechanism, the Foundation can then fund an expansion to see if the program will be effective in other geographical areas or if variations of the program will affect its impact.

An early example is emergency medical services. In the 1970s, there was no 911 to call in a medical emergency. Individual cities and counties had their own emergency numbers, or a person in need simply dialed an operator, who would dispatch an ambulance. Terry Keenan and other members of the early Foundation staff knew about the emergency medical system in Connecticut—the nation's first. In fact, The Commonwealth Fund, Keenan's previous employer, had given a grant to Jack Cole, the chairman of surgery at the Yale School of Medicine, to improve trauma care in Connecticut. Keenan also knew Blair Sadler, who had helped launch the New Haven emergency medical services program. The Foundation then funded an expansion of the Connecticut program in a number of regions and recruited Sadler as a vice president to run it. "What the Robert Wood Johnson Foundation did was to take that concept and multiply it nationwide in about fifty-four regions," Keenan recalled in a 1997 interview for the Foundation's oral history.

AIDS provides another example of the Foundation staff seeking and acting upon the advice of others as it used its own expertise to develop a program. As the AIDS epidemic spread across the country in the 1980s, with no treatment in sight, the Foundation began thinking about what it could do to prevent HIV and care for people with AIDS. Drew Altman, at the time a Foundation vice president, read a magazine story about what San Francisco was doing to treat AIDS patients. Altman called Phil Lee, who was president of the San Francisco Health Commission, and asked him to set up a visit for him and Paul Jellinek, who was a senior program officer at the Foundation at that time and who later became a vice president. Altman and Jellinek flew to San Francisco to see the program firsthand.

"Obviously, the conditions in San Francisco were unusual in that you had a politically effective gay community; you had a surplus in the public health budget; and you had some very good leadership in the health department," Jellinek recalls. "But could the San Francisco approach work in a place like Miami or New Orleans or Atlanta or Jersey City—or wherever?" Foundation President Rogers invited Lee and Mervyn Silverman, the San Francisco public health director, to Princeton to talk with the Foundation's staff and Board about its community-based approach to preventing AIDS and caring for HIV-positive people. They were so persuasive that the Foundation funded replications of the San Francisco model in eleven communities. Congress adopted the approach when it passed the Ryan White Act in 1990.

A third example is the Community Programs for Affordable Health Care. In the early 1980s, a widely publicized program in Rochester, New York, came to the attention of the Foundation's program staff. To save health care costs, leading Rochester businesses—Eastman Kodak and Xerox among them—formed an alliance to provide more efficient care to their employees by establishing a multifaceted approach including health planning, expansions of health maintenance organizations, and hospital revenue caps. To see if the model would be effective in other places, the Foundation, having consulted with business leaders in Rochester, funded an expansion of the concept in eleven additional locations. An evaluation concluded that the program did not work, largely because the levers to lower health care costs existed at the federal and state levels, rather than the local level.

### Open Calls for Proposals

Although most of the Foundation's calls for proposals are targeted attempts to replicate what already seems to be a good idea, some calls for proposals are open and have relatively loose criteria; they identify a problem and ask applicants to come up with solutions.

The AIDS Prevention and Services Program, the second of the Foundation's AIDS programs, is an example of this approach. "I remember sitting in the cafeteria at lunch," Jellinek recalls, "and I said to Lee Cluff, who was the Foundation's president at the time, 'Lee, what if we were to just put a different kind of call for proposals together... We just say, Send us your best ideas for AIDS prevention.'" Cluff liked the idea, and the Foundation sent out an open call for proposals along the lines Jellinek had suggested. The response was huge. More than one thousand organizations submitted applications, and the applications were diverse in approach, location, and population served.

A variation of this approach is the Robert Wood Johnson Foundation Local Funding Partnerships Program, which was previously called the Local Initiative Funding Partners Program. The brainchild of Terry Keenan, who in his travels had observed the many good ideas that germinated in local communities, the program offered state and community foundations the opportunity to submit interesting proposals to the Robert Wood Johnson Foundation. Both the sponsoring local foundations and the

Robert Wood Johnson Foundation would then fund successful applicants. At first, the Foundation was very prescriptive, setting out rigorous guidelines and limits that the local foundations had to follow. Gradually, however, the Foundation staff learned that they would get more creative proposals by reducing restrictions and opening up the process.

### Investigator-Initiated Ideas

In the late 1970s, David Olds, a newly minted PhD, had a big idea. He believed that if public health nurses were able to advise young, low-income, first-time pregnant women during the last part of their pregnancies and through their babies' infancy, it would improve the ability of the mothers to raise their children and, ultimately, improve the children's health. He brought to the Robert Wood Johnson Foundation his idea of a trial program in Elmira, New York, located in a rural county of about one hundred thousand people. Program officers remember being impressed with both the experiment's scientific design and the fact that it had sound theoretical underpinnings, and the Foundation agreed to fund it. An evaluation deemed it to be successful.

The Foundation next funded a second trial in Memphis to see whether the approach would work in an urban environment. Subsequently, the Nurse-Family Partnership program took off—to such an extent that funding for nurse home visitation programs, such as the Nurse-Family Partnership, was included in the Affordable Care Act.

That was an example of a program's having been brought to the Foundation's attention by a potential grantee by way of an over-the-transom request. Another such program was the National Center on Addiction and Substance Abuse at Columbia University, which Joseph Califano, the former Secretary of Health, Education, and Welfare, suggested to Steven Schroeder not long after Schroeder became the Foundation's president.

From 1972 until 2003, the Foundation had a policy to accept and review all proposals that met minimal criteria standards submitted to it. "We used to spend a lot of time reviewing unsolicited proposals," recalls Jellinek. "In fact, though national programs rarely came from these, we awarded many grants to individuals on the basis of their over-the-transom solicitations."

Although this policy was meant to be an open-sourcing mechanism for getting ideas from a wide range of people, it was largely abandoned as the Foundation became more intentionally strategic in the early 2000s. From 2008 on, with the exception of the pioneer portfolio, the Foundation considered only proposals that came to it in response to a specific solicitation. By contrast, the pioneer portfolio found accepting unsolicited proposals valuable. "The yield is very small; we fund only two or three projects per year from the hundreds that come across the transom," says Brian Quinn, a former leader of the pioneer team. "But it's an important way to find new ideas."

### Building on Foundation Programs as a Model for Similar Ones

It is not uncommon for staff members to seek program ideas from within the Foundation itself; that is, to take the core of an existing program and develop a similar one in a new or related field.

The Tobacco Policy Research and Evaluation Program offers a good example. Research from this program demonstrated that raising tobacco taxes and enacting clean indoor air laws decreased smoking by young people. Recognizing the effectiveness of policy research, the Foundation expanded its scope from tobacco to alcohol and drug abuse by developing the Substance Abuse Policy Research Program. After the Foundation designated reducing childhood obesity as a priority, it developed research programs to examine the policy and environmental factors that would increase healthy eating and physical activity.

On an even broader level, the Foundation's approach to reducing childhood obesity was patterned substantially on its experience in reducing smoking. The Foundation's tobacco-control programming combined policy research, advocacy, demonstration programs, and communications campaigns, and the programming to reduce childhood obesity took a similar approach.

Another model was the Clinical Scholars Program, which trained physicians in social science research and leadership skills. Later it spawned programs to train professors to teach and research health finance; nurses to do clinical research; dentists to do health services research; economists, sociologists, and political scientists to do research on health issues; and scholars to turn their attention to population health. This model dominated the Foundation's work in developing human capital for its first forty years.

In summary, the traditional way in which the Foundation found ideas and developed programs depended largely on the experience and expertise of the staff, which developed priorities and program directions in consultation with knowledgeable people in the field.

## —⟋⟍— Finding Ideas 3: The Pioneer Way

The pioneer portfolio represents an attempt to open the Foundation to new ideas and innovative thinkers. It was established to operate like a venture capital fund—one that was expected to find and invest in bold, transformative ideas, most of which would fail in practice but some of which would succeed wildly. As the staff told the Board, the purpose of the pioneer portfolio was to "promote a culture that values experimentation and unconventional approaches."

And how would the pioneer portfolio do that? In an early meeting of the pioneer team, Lewis Sandy, the Foundation's executive vice president at the time, asked the members what they wanted to do with this opportunity. He listened to the responses for nearly the entire meeting, concluding that they wanted to swing for the fences and not be bound by convention.

Probably the most important step in creating a new culture, according to Steve Downs, who became a leader of the pioneer team and is now the Foundation's chief technology and information officer, was deciding not to make any grants in the first year. Instead, the time was used to discuss potential projects and explain why they would be pioneering. In addition, the pioneer team wanted to learn from similar philanthropic efforts, such as The Pew Charitable Trusts' Venture Fund and the James Irvine Foundation's Arts Innovation Fund, both of which had been judged unsuccessful by their own foundations. After interviewing people involved in those efforts, Downs and Chinwe Onyekere, a program associate at the time, concluded that the pioneer team had to be knowledgeable, fast, and nimble—but also rigorous.

"Pioneer," said Downs in 2004, "is about creating the environment for ideas, bringing fresh minds to problems—even looking outside health and health care—and being able to recognize potential. These kinds of changes will involve a lot of trial and error, and we are comfortable with that. But it is a change of mindset for us to be able to look at work that has a reasonably high chance of failure and say 'Let's go for it.'"[5]

### New Networks

Pioneer's main way of finding new ideas has been by tapping into networks of innovators and entrepreneurs. "The bulk of our work is through our networks," says Paul Tarini, a former leader of the pioneer team, "through the people we know and the people they know." This means that the pioneer team members must constantly build, strengthen, and foster their networks. "If networks are not sufficiently big or diverse," says Brian Quinn, "we start running into groupthink and don't generate new ideas."

In this way, Lynn Etheredge, a leading thinker on rapid learning and a Foundation grantee, led pioneer team members to David Eddy, who had an idea for a project called the Archimedes Healthcare Simulator (ARCHeS) that used data to simulate the impact of various changes on health care. Impressed by Eddy's idea, the Foundation funded the Archimedes Simulator.

To gain access to networks of innovators, the pioneer team funded meetings where innovators gathered. Initially, pioneer funded TED and then TEDMED meetings to explore innovative ideas.* It was at TEDMED that Tarini met Jamie Heywood of *PatientsLikeMe*, which the Foundation later funded. A TED conference became the place where the Foundation discovered Thomas Goetz, the founder of Iodine, a San Francisco-based health technology company. Goetz, who became the entrepreneur-in-residence at the Foundation during 2013 and 2014, helped develop Flip the Clinic, a clearinghouse for what works and what doesn't in the doctor-patient encounter.

Michael Painter, a senior program officer, heard Salman Khan, the founder of Khan Academy, speak about its approach to education at TED. After the talk, Painter discussed potential collaboration with Shantanu Sinha, the president and chief operating officer of Khan Academy. The effort is leading to Khan Academy's creation of video content to help students prepare for the Medical College Admission Test.

To develop other networks, the Foundation, upon the pioneer team's recommendation, funded O'Reilly Media to develop the 2011 Health Foo (Friends of O'Reilly) Camp. Health Foo Camp allowed for unstructured, free-ranging discussions of potential solutions to problems in health and health care. It also offered opportunities to network. Those networking opportunities led the Foundation to make grants to the Data & Society Research Institute to hold a conference on Big Data and to Creative Commons to collect and use real-time data from people to improve health.

---

* TED (Technology, Education, Design) is a global set of conferences to foster the spread of great ideas. Owned by The Sapling Foundation, TED aims to provide a platform for the world's smartest thinkers, greatest visionaries, and most-inspiring teachers, so that millions of people can gain a better understanding of the biggest issues faced by the world, and feed a desire to help create a better future. TEDMED focuses on health and medicine.

## Prize Philanthropy

Prizes have long been a way to spur innovation. Back in 1795, Napoleon Bonaparte offered 12,000 francs to anyone who invented a food-preservation technique that would help feed his troops. One Nicolas Appert, a French confectioner, invented SPAM—the food, not the Internet annoyance—and walked off with the prize.[6] In the twentieth century, one of the best-known prizes was the $25,000 Orteig Prize, offered by New York hotel owner Raymond Orteig to the first person to fly nonstop between New York and Paris. Charles Lindbergh took the prize money in 1927. More recently, to encourage commercial space flight, the XPrize (now the Ansari XPrize) offered $10 million to the first nongovernmental organization to launch a reusable manned spacecraft into space twice within two weeks. The prize was won in 2004 by Scaled Composites, a company financed by Microsoft cofounder Paul Allen, which built and launched SpaceShipOne. The America COMPETES Reauthorization ACT of 2010 allows federal agencies to use prizes to spur innovation.

The pioneer team worked with the XPRIZE Foundation to design projects that would spur smoking cessation and end obesity. It decided, however, not to go forward with either XPrize. "We didn't think the systems were in place to support a prize," says Chinwe Onyekere, who at the time was the Foundation's program officer for the XPrize. "The problem was verifying whether participants actually did what they said they did, such as to quit smoking and stay off cigarettes for two years. It would take many layers of auditing to determine if the prize had been won."[7]

Although the XPrize didn't receive funding, the Foundation did support two other types of prize philanthropy. One was Ashoka Changemakers' Disruptive Innovations in Health and Health Care competition. Through the six competitions it supported, the Foundation discovered three projects that it agreed to fund: Project ECHO, in which specialists share information with primary care providers in underserved areas (this program was the subject of an *Anthology* chapter in volume XIV); Family Coaching Clinics, which were mental health clinics modeled after pharmacy mini-clinics; and Asociaçâo Saude Crianca, a Brazilian organization that addresses health through antipoverty programs.

In the other prize competition, the pioneer team funded HopeLab to hold the *Ruckus Nation* prize for the best idea to encourage physical activity among middle school students. The competition received 429 entries. In 2008, Stacy Cho, a middle school teacher from Seattle, won the $50,000 grand prize with *Dancing Craze*, an interactive game with wearable motion sensors.

### Pitch Day

In 2013, as another way to stimulate new approaches to improve health and health care, the pioneer team organized Pitch Day. The team sent out a call for proposals with the potential to transform health and health care, and a panel of judges selected eight of the 521 proposals. The eight finalists then went to New York City in October 2013 and pitched their ideas to the judges, the purpose being not only to seek Foundation funding, but also to interest other investors in these ideas. Pioneer team members expect the Foundation to fund several of them.

### Innovations Adopted from Other Fields

The pioneer team has also been interested in taking successful innovations in one field and applying them to another. For example, Lori Melichar, director of pioneer team, wrote that the team "engaged in a five-year behavioral economics initiative because applying an emerging—or even a well-established—perspective from another field has the potential to uncover game-changing insights that can generate traction in health and health care."[8]

Behavioral economics uses psychology to understand and change economic behavior by "nudging" people. The Foundation has funded studies examining incentives to increase the use of advance directives, immunizations, and physical activity among older adults. It also funded research to test colored labels indicating the healthiness of food choices in cafeterias—green for healthy foods, yellow for less healthy foods, and red for unhealthy foods. This traffic-light labeling helped consumers make healthier food choices. Another behavioral economics study found that the best way to increase flu vaccination rates among college students is with small financial incentives. Studies under way in 2014 are focused on reducing the use of low-value tests and procedures by providers.

In another adoption of an idea, "prediction markets," which aggregate traders' purchases into a crowdsourced prediction of an event, has been broadened from politics and business to health. The Iowa Electronic Markets (IEM), for example, conducts futures trading to predict presidential and other elections. Since prediction markets are good predictors of elections, why couldn't they be used to predict infectious disease trends? Under a grant recommended by the pioneer team, IEM conducted markets on predicting both seasonal flu and swine flu. Markets for seasonal flu and swine flu accurately forecast the spread of those diseases.

## —∾— Finding Ideas 4: The Present and Near Future

In retrospect, the greatest contribution of the pioneer portfolio has been that it opened the Foundation to ideas and networks beyond the health world.[†] Although the pioneer team did not consider itself limited to technology, many ideas discovered by the team

---

[†] It should be noted that the pioneer team does not have a monopoly on seeking ideas from innovators. The vulnerable populations team, for example, funded the Green House program, a smaller and gentler kind of nursing home, based on the staff's meeting its founder, Bill Thomas, a geriatrician who had previously tried to change the culture of nursing homes with the Eden Alternative.

involved technologies such as video games and electronic medical records.

That thinking—exploring beyond the walls of the Foundation and of health—permeated the strategic planning process the Foundation carried out in 2013. The group charged with developing a strategic plan consciously explored what was happening in areas such as behavioral health and statistical analysis (Big Data) that could be used to improve health and health care. To be sure that it understood plausible scenarios for the future, the Foundation invited leading thinkers to explore trends in their fields.

Now that the Foundation has adopted a new vision—advancing a culture of health—and is developing implementation plans, how is it going about getting ideas and developing new programs? By and large, it is through the traditional use of the expertise of the staff and the outside experts the staff consults. In developing new strategic directions and implementation plans, the staff relies on its own knowledge and experience, even as it consults with leading experts. Indeed, there is no substitute for the curiosity, experience, and judgment found in the best Foundation program officers—who have always relied on their own sources and networks for ideas.

There has been one major change, however. The Foundation is now reaching out to people beyond its own fields in search of new ideas. It has invited historians, economists, and social scientists to tell the staff about the latest developments in their fields. Thus, the approach adopted by the pioneer team has, to an extent, permeated the way the Foundation as a whole does business; it is more open to ideas from the outside than it had been in the past. Moreover, the Foundation is exploring what other foundations and businesses are doing so that it neither acts in isolation nor duplicates activities that others are carrying out.

With all the changes, is there a role left for the individual prospectors for ideas—the Terry Keenans of the world? Or are they like the small corner bookstore—something that existed in the past but no longer has a place in the world of Amazon?

Just as there still seems to be a place for a Strand bookstore in New York City or a Powell's bookstore in Portland, Oregon, there should be a place for the Terry Keenans. Such seekers will not replace the Internet or the networks of big thinkers, but they can be invaluable in finding new and creative ideas. After all, good ideas can come from anywhere, and it is a foundation's role to develop all of its capacities to recognize and exploit them.

## Notes

1. Quoted in M. Lewis, *The New New Thing* (Norton: New York, 2000), 251.
2. S. Johnson, *Where Good Ideas Come From* (Riverhead Books: New York, 2010), 221.
3. J. Surowiecki, *The Wisdom of Crowds: Why the Many Are Smarter Than the Few and How Collective Wisdom Shapes Business, Societies, and Nations* (Doubleday: New York, 2004), 31–32.
4. T. Proscio, "The Pioneer Portfolio," in this volume, Chapter 2.
5. "The Pioneer Portfolio: A New Initiative," *RWJF Advances*, Issue I, 2004, 4.
6. P. Nowak, *Sex, Bombs and Burgers* (Guilford, CT: Lyons Press, 2011), 55.
7. "An X Prize for Health and Health Care: RWJF Explores the Idea," RWJF Program Results Report, http://www.rwjf.org/reports/grr/057761.html.
8. http://www.rwjf.org/en/blogs/pioneering-ideas/2013/05/search_for_pioneerin.html.

# The Pioneer Portfolio

*Tony Proscio*

## Introduction

Shortly after becoming the president and CEO of the Robert Wood Johnson Foundation in 2003, Risa Lavizzo-Mourey began the development of an "Impact Framework" to guide the organization's future grantmaking. The Impact Framework established a number of portfolios in areas of high priority to the Foundation, such as expanding health insurance coverage, improving services to vulnerable populations, and reducing childhood obesity. It also set up an entirely new "pioneer portfolio"—one that was expected to be nimble in responding to emerging opportunities and to take chances on new, breakthrough ideas that could change health and health care. The development of the pioneer portfolio, the staff told the Board, "marks the first time that the Foundation has deliberately and distinctly recognized the opportunity to pursue new ventures that are expected to represent a different approach to grantmaking."

More than ten years out, it is appropriate to look back and see how the pioneer portfolio has gone about its work and what it has accomplished. In this chapter, Tony Proscio offers a retrospective report on the pioneer portfolio. He examines the way in which the pioneer team sought out new ideas and innovators; discusses some of the projects that the pioneer portfolio nurtured; and assesses the pros and cons of establishing a separate unit within a foundation to find and support innovations.

To the best our knowledge, only two other foundations in the health field have created a unit charged specifically with looking for groundbreaking ideas. One of them, The California HealthCare Foundation, has taken a somewhat different approach from that of the Robert Wood Johnson Foundation. Somewhat like a venture capital firm, it invests in a limited number of companies that it believes have the potential to develop breakthroughs in improving healthcare. The Commonwealth Fund recently established its own innovations unit, based partly on the Robert Wood Johnson Foundation model.

An author, journalist, and strategic planning consultant, Tony Proscio is a senior fellow at the Center for Strategic Philanthropy and Civil Society at Duke University's Sanford School of Public Policy and a consultant to foundations and major nonprofit organizations. He has written frequently for the *Anthology* series.

—ɯ— Nearly all foundations innovate. Or at least they try
to. Admittedly, the definition of "innovation" varies from place to
place—a better way of delivering a traditional service may count
as innovation to one pair of eyes; someone else may reserve the
term only for changes that would replace the service altogether,
upending the very idea of what the service was meant to accomplish. Still, whether they seek incremental or radical change, many
foundations will say—sometimes on the first page of their annual
reports—that one of their chief products is innovation.

It has become a kind of industry proverb that philanthropy is
the research-and-development arm of society. But that poses some
corollary questions: If foundations are supposed to be the labora-
tories of social, scientific, and cultural invention, where do *their*
new ideas come from? And what keeps foundations from sinking,
over time, into intellectual and technological ruts?

On this, there are two broad schools of thought. The
predominant view is that the ability to discern and weigh new
ideas comes from deep expertise in one's field—accumulated
experience and knowledge, years of firsthand inquiry and
experimentation, the patient harvest of the concentrated mind.
Following that principle, many foundations hire staff members
who are considered "content experts"—people with academic
training, frontline experience, and distinguished reputations in
the foundation's fields of choice. Or foundations may recruit
generalists for their own staff but then forge close relationships
with content experts among their grantees.

However they choose to do it, foundation managers typically
rely on the content experts to scan the horizons of their discipline,
locating and testing the new ideas that will propel the field into
the future. If they feel a rut beginning to form, they may simply
recruit new experts or change the category of problems on which
they choose to work.

A different, less common view is that profound innovation requires a degree of detachment from normal expert circles. According to this view, the tight professional networks of deep expertise can sometimes form a wall of insulation against radically new approaches—the kinds of big breakthroughs that management theorist Clayton Christensen labeled "disruptive." To pursue that type of innovation, some managers believe they need teams that aren't steeped in a single discipline, technology, or strategic mindset and aren't part of the institution's normal production routines.

To take an example from the tech industry, think of the shift from hard disk drives to flash memory. As Clayton Christensen described it in his influential 1997 book *The Innovator's Dilemma*, leading hard disk manufacturers of the mid-1990s had all the expertise they would have needed to enter and dominate the flash-drive market.[1] But their senior executives, and the executives' network of suppliers and customers, weren't much interested in flash drives, which they viewed as simply an inferior variation on hard disks. And so the companies neglected the new technology—until other firms, untethered to the habits of hard disk customers, envisioned and ultimately tapped completely different pools of demand, revolutionizing how a growing percentage of the world's data is stored.

One might imagine that foundations, following this line of reasoning, would conclude that the big innovations—the ideas that change how problems are defined and solved—need to be nurtured among people who are not enmeshed in the intellectual circuitry of established programs, strategies, and methods. But it's rare to see that view reflected in the organization charts of major foundations. Several have set aside funds, and occasionally staff positions, for activities that fall outside their official priorities. But in most cases, these separate units aren't charged with prospecting for new—much less revolutionary—ideas. Instead, they usually manage projects that don't fit the rest of the institution's work but are deemed important for other reasons. The vast majority of

American foundations, judging from their structure and staffing patterns, remain committed to deep expertise, not only as a way of managing current programs but also as a primary source for new ideas and insights.

## —᠊ᠳᠠ— The Search for Innovation at the Robert Wood Johnson Foundation

For most of its forty-one-year history, the Robert Wood Johnson Foundation has been a near-textbook case of philanthropy built on deep expertise. Its focus on health and health care has placed it squarely within fields such as medicine, public health, and research, in which specialization is prized and professional or scholarly distinction is a prerequisite for any kind of leadership. Consequently, the Foundation's program staff is heavy with people who have devoted their careers, and made significant contributions, to one or more of these fields. But in the early 2000s, some Foundation officers began asking if there were other ways of organizing the search for new ideas. Might a new kind of team be able to uncover more radical kinds of innovation—approaches that would be unlikely to spring naturally from the traditional wells of expertise?

Specifically, it was around the turn of the millennium that the idea of disruptive innovation, influenced partly by Christensen's book, became a theme of what one early innovator at the Foundation, then vice president Robert G. Hughes, describes as "a series of discussions, brainstorming sessions, ideas bandied about over lunch." This line of thinking surfaced during a time of organizational ferment throughout the Foundation, as a new strategic plan was being implemented and grantmaking teams were being reorganized under a health group and a health care group. By 2001, the newly appointed Foundation senior vice president and director of the health care group, Risa Lavizzo-Mourey, was joining in some of these disruptive-innovation discussions, and she encouraged Hughes to distill the strongest ideas into a proposal.

The result, in July of that year, was an internal concept paper titled "The Pioneer Portfolio: A Pilot Project."

The paper opened with the observation that "The health care group teams, while at different stages, all have a strong complement of program staff with depth and expertise, as well as several years of experience working together. [However] ... projects intended to help the Group consider *future* strategic areas that a new team could target are not within the purview of the current teams." The premise of the paper, as Hughes later summarized it, was that the more an institution focuses on particular goals, and the more it is devoted to them, the less opportunity there is for other kinds of innovation and new ideas to emerge.

Hughes recommended that the health care group create a new team—one that, like a new business development unit in the private sector, could reach outside the group's established priorities, respond rapidly to new trends and opportunities, absorb higher risk, and focus primarily on the potential effects of big or unexpected changes in health care. Yet, despite keeping its sights trained on the field's far horizons, its essential purpose would be "research and development for the health care group"—a scouting operation, in effect, for future Foundation programs in health care.

Slightly more than a year after Hughes submitted the paper, Lavizzo-Mourey became the Foundation's president and CEO. Among her earliest decisions was to expand the idea of a pioneer portfolio from solely a health care group initiative to a Foundation-wide innovation unit. In July 2003, Lavizzo-Mourey introduced the Impact Framework, which outlined the Foundation's overall grantmaking approach and structure. It established four program portfolios: vulnerable populations, human capital, a cluster of initiatives targeted on specific health and health care challenges, and pioneer. As conceived at the time, the pioneer portfolio's purpose would be to uncover promising new ideas that other teams and programs could explore and adopt. The pioneer team was charged with seeking and supporting "innovative ideas and approaches across a broad spectrum of topics in the health and health care fields." Hughes, who was soon named the Foundation's chief learning officer, initially kept pioneer under his purview, thus ensuring its insulation from the other three program groups.

The pioneer budget was by far the smallest of the four portfolios—less than 1 percent of the Foundation's total grant-making at the start, and around 5 percent in later years—but it had the broadest mandate and the greatest scope for exploration. Significantly, the description of its mandate in the impact framework, and in later documents, did not emphasize finding new initiatives for the other groups and teams. Rather than a traditional R&D unit, limited solely to incubating future activity for mainstream adoption, pioneer would be free to explore whole new fields and disciplines, weave networks of its own, and pursue ideas even if they were, for the moment, wholly unrelated to other goals, strategies, programs, and priorities. The only limitation was that the purpose of any project must be, in some way, to improve health and health care in the United States.

In fact, the team was not merely free to explore broadly; it was virtually mandated to do so. As Lavizzo-Mourey put it recently, reflecting on her thinking at the time, "If you look at big discoveries, groundbreaking discoveries, they often come about when people from fields that don't usually interact come together. Take the double helix, for example: physics and biology. Philanthropy has that potential. But you have to really want to find those innovations that are outside of where you would usually look, because they are being developed in a region that is not central to your own field."

## —⚹— A Culture within a Culture

Pioneer's program staff, consistently numbering in the single digits, has been drawn mostly from other Foundation teams, and most pioneer members spend part of their time working on other, more narrowly focused portfolios. Between 2003 and 2013, the team made roughly $200 million in grants for explorations on the far periphery of health philanthropy. Unlike most other teams, pioneer welcomes unsolicited proposals; it prides itself on having bankrolled some ideas that arrived unbidden. Its work has occasionally touched on themes of direct interest to other teams, but most of it has been so dissimilar to that of other Foundation programs and portfolios that some staff members—both inside and outside the pioneer team—have sometimes asked themselves what connects pioneer to the rest of the Foundation, other than its address.

The answer to that question has changed over time and has always entailed what Hughes calls an "ongoing creative tension." The goal in establishing an innovation unit, he says, was to ensure that it wasn't so restrained by Foundation priorities and preoccupations that it might miss something important taking place elsewhere, with important implications for health and health care. Even so, he has been careful to say from the outset that pioneer was not meant to be a "skunk works"—a freewheeling group of employees working in a hothouse atmosphere, deliberately insulated from the rest of the company, exempt from most management constraints, and charged with inventing unimagined new things. (The colorful term *skunk works*, widely used in industry, comes from a trademarked division of Lockheed Martin that was originally formed to create a new fighter jet in World War II.)

Pioneer *was* meant to be different from the rest of the institution—both in content and in style. "One of the images we came back to from time to time," says Hughes, "was that of a spaceship in orbit: wanting to hit that perfect spot, beyond gravity but still orbiting the earth, while staying connected to all the other work the Foundation does, and taking advantage of these huge resources, all those networks, all those connections, all that experience of thirty-some years, and the reputation the

Foundation had established. The challenge was how to take advantage of that without getting drawn into a particular way of thinking so much that we weren't open to new ideas."

An early and longstanding pioneer project illustrates how the team initially struck that balance in its first few years. Among the staff's first avenues of exploration was the explosion of data on all aspects of life, including medicine and health, and the corresponding growth of technology to make data more widely available and usable. Studying burgeoning datasets drawn from science and health care, the team noticed that one interesting and seemingly important gap was the kind of data that capture people's day-to-day experiences (such as diet, sleep, pain, moods, and physical activity), and connects that information with their health. It seemed that if patients started keeping such personal records electronically, not only could they monitor and manage their own health better, but they would also begin building a national database that researchers and clinicians could use to spot patterns and draw broader conclusions.

After a couple of years spent probing the field and contacting networks of people exploring new ideas in health data, the pioneer team joined forces with the California HealthCare Foundation. In 2006, the two foundations jointly made grants to eight interdisciplinary teams to start designing applications. On its own, the pioneer team then supported four more teams in subsequent rounds. The goal was to create ways for patients to record their observations of daily living in relatively standard personal health records. Later, grantees set out to test whether these new records could be used to improve the quality of care and the patients' resulting health. The effort, called Project HealthDesign, eventually amounted to roughly $10 million in pioneer investments.

The connection with the Foundation's mission and current interests is easy to see. Not only did Project HealthDesign aim squarely at the intersection between health and health care, it also hoped to improve the quality of care patients receive—an explicit goal of one of the Foundation's targeted programs. Yet Project HealthDesign did not emerge from, or even significantly involve, the team working on quality. It arose from connections carefully formed by Steve Downs, the pioneer team's first team leader and currently the Foundation's chief technology and information officer, among people exploring the possible uses of personal health records and user-generated data to improve health.

Besides exploring technical questions such as which data to gather and what kind of interface and platform to create, the researchers also used the Foundation's support to examine legal and moral questions involved in collecting people's personal information. One consequence of the ongoing work, Downs believes, has been to bridge the intellectual divide between what had been early-stage work in the day-to-day collection of user data and the more advanced field of health care informatics.

By itself, Project HealthDesign probably didn't detonate an explosive breakthrough in the collection and use of personal health data—at least it hasn't yet. But it has drawn attention and energy to a field that would likely have gathered steam much more slowly, if at all. In any case, creating a revolutionary breakthrough with every project isn't the real goal of pioneer grantmaking. Much of the team's effort is devoted to developing relationships and inter-disciplinary connections, both to advance particular ideas and to help fertilize the broader terrain on which new ideas might grow. From the rich mix of explorations and inquiries, they reason, some promising ideas might gain momentum (fueled partly by the legit-imacy that comes with recognition by the Foundation), and addi-tional possibilities for breakthroughs may spring up. "Every ven-ture capitalist hopes that one investment will turn out to be a Facebook," Downs says. "I think the idea is analogous here; we pursue a lot of things, trying to find a few that make a fundamen-tal change."

## —∿— Networking the Networks

Another advantage of forging relationships with a wide range of innovative people and infiltrating their networks is that these connections tend to lead to more and more new possibilities. This happened, for example, in the development of a project that ultimately became one of the pioneer team's most promising. Known as Project ECHO (Extension for Community Healthcare Outcomes), it uses communication technology to bring specialists in chronic or complex diseases, who tend to be based in large metropolitan hospitals, into contact with physicians and nurses treating these diseases in remote rural areas. Project ECHO is essentially a long-distance but intimate professional education program for health care providers who would otherwise never have access to such advanced learning.[2]

The Foundation's relationship with Project ECHO did not spring from a pioneer effort to find better ways of educating clinicians, or even from a search for new applications for communication technology. It came from one contact recommending another contact, leading to a chain of connections.

Around the time of the pioneer portfolio's launch, Nancy Barrand, then a Foundation senior program officer and currently a senior adviser for program development, was reading a book about social entrepreneurs worldwide. Most of the people featured in the book had been sponsored by an organization called Ashoka: Innovators for the Public, which marshals venture capital for such entrepreneurs. Coincidentally, Barrand was also consulting with an outside adviser on ways of raising capital for innovations in the health sector, and he had suggested contacting Ashoka. Barrand invited Bill Drayton, Ashoka's founder, to speak to her Foundation colleagues. This ultimately led to the Foundation's making a grant to Ashoka to explore new ways of financing social entrepreneurship in health.

As a result of that relationship, Barrand became acquainted with another of Ashoka's programs, called Changemakers, which sponsors competitions to find innovative solutions to social problems. Here, she thought, might be one model for how pioneer could cast a wider net in seeking possible recipients for its grants. Working with Ashoka, the pioneer team devised a competition called Disruptive Innovations in Health and Health Care, which drew a large number of responses. Among the winning submissions in the first round of that competition was Project ECHO, which at that point was a one-state pilot project funded by state and federal grants, focusing on treating hepatitis C in New Mexico.

Invited to submit a fuller proposal to pioneer for final consideration, Project ECHO responded modestly, with only a request to evaluate its current activities. This struck Barrand and her colleagues as small-bore. Among other things, the proposal gave the impression of a local boutique undertaking, without significant national implications. Viewed from far away, it seemed to some people like little more than routine telemedicine—a useful technology but not especially groundbreaking. But Barrand's interest had been piqued by the project's initial contest submission. Sensing an undeveloped opportunity, she set off to visit Project ECHO's home base at the University of Mexico in Albuquerque and view it up close.

There, Barrand asked founder Sanjeev Arora, a highly regarded gastroenterologist, to set aside his proposal and simply describe how Project ECHO could change ongoing professional education in health care around the world. That was, of course, too big an undertaking for the Robert Wood Johnson Foundation to fund on its own, but it gave Arora a signal he hadn't heard before: someone was interested in pursuing his *real* vision. He hadn't dared to write the full concept into his proposal, he told Barrand, because he believed the Foundation—any foundation, for that matter—would consider it pie in the sky. He was mistaken.

"There was something there," Barrand recalls, "something fundamental in Project ECHO, which is why they had won. And it was the central, core concept of de-monopolizing knowledge."

Within half a dozen years, pioneer's support for Project ECHO has amounted to more than $10 million, including a new national institute focused on replicating the project nationwide. Arora has gone on to raise additional support from national funders and federal agencies, and has begun working with foreign governments on international replication.

The story is unique in many ways, but it illustrates a basic pattern that has become close to routine at pioneer—one innovator introduces a staff member to another innovator; the staff member introduces other staff members; other connections follow, and somewhere along the chain of encounters, an opportunity begins to flower.

## —⁓— Harnessing the Power of Data

Another example of this pattern—and an especially rich source of overlapping networks and serendipitous connections—has been the explosion of Big Data. Under that giant conceptual tent lie many fields of information gathering that specifically relate to health, including the many ways that people are collecting data on their own activities and conditions (think of wireless trackers that monitor exercise, sleep, and heart rate, or glucose monitors for diabetics), that health care providers are collecting data on their services and patients, and that corporations are collecting data on their products and customers. Much of this information pours into databases hour by hour or day by day, constantly aggregating more and more information on behavior, health, use of services and medicines, and the relationships among all these things. As the variety and quality of the data grows, the number of possible uses multiplies. And so does the constellation of fields and experts who might be enlisted in the search for ideas.

The pioneer team had a toe in these waters relatively early in its history, thanks to Project HealthDesign. Team members were also exploring farther afield, attending conferences and consulting with experts on the data explosion, sensing that somewhere in this still-inchoate universe, or perhaps in several places, ideas were simmering that might lead to something genuinely disruptive.

Meanwhile on another, mostly unrelated track—having less to do with Big Data than fast data—the team was exploring ways that electronic communication could accelerate the pace at which information reaches scholars, health care institutions, practitioners, and patients. For example, an early project in this category of work, called Rapid Learning, sought to build a nationwide system of databases that could unlock information on new technologies and treatments and deliver it more quickly to researchers and clinicians.[3]

Lynn Etheredge, the architect of Rapid Learning, had assembled a circle of advisers and industry experts to help think through the technical opportunities and challenges. One of them was David Eddy, founder of Archimedes, Inc., a company that had developed a sophisticated proprietary set of algorithms for combining vast amounts of data and hundreds of equations to create simulated clinical trials. The Archimedes Model essentially makes it possible for medical researchers, when carrying out research on a wide range of diseases and conditions, to avoid recruiting volunteers, creating and maintaining control groups, and tackling the many complexities of experiments with human subjects. With data from hundreds of thousands of actual (but anonymous) medical records, certain kinds of questions can be answered with considerable precision, and far more quickly than through a standard clinical trial.

At Etheredge's request, Eddy had written a concept paper on how Archimedes might put some of its mastery of data management, computing, and modeling to use in advancing the Rapid Learning project. From that paper, and in conversations with Etheredge and Eddy, Nancy Barrand began to envision far wider access to the Archimedes Model itself—making its analytical and experimental power available to vastly more users, including discounted rates for public policymakers and nonprofit health organizations that normally couldn't afford the standard fee for

Archimedes' services. Extending their growing relationship with Rapid Learning to a new one with Archimedes, pioneer members started negotiating what later became a $15.6 million grant to create ARCHeS, short for Archimedes Health Care Simulator. It is a comparatively simple online tool that lets researchers and policy analysts conduct quick inquiries into health care questions and compare the cost and effectiveness of different treatment scenarios.[4]

The ARCHeS story isn't simply another example of one point on a network leading to another. It also illustrates the unconventional approach to grantmaking taken by the pioneer team. Archimedes is a for-profit company, roughly twenty years old, with strong prospects for growth, that is a subsidiary of Kaiser Permanente, a nonprofit health care organization. While making a grant to such an enterprise is far from unheard of, it is quite complicated. Most obviously, the Foundation needed to ensure that the grant would be used solely for purposes consistent with its charitable mission. In this case, that meant ensuring that ARCHeS would make the Archimedes technology widely available to nonprofits and government at discounted rates for many years. But there were subtler complexities, too: Archimedes is a growing and fast-changing enterprise. What if it were sold or otherwise changed owners? What if it ran into financial trouble or went out of business? These questions took years to work through.

Unlike other Foundation teams, the pioneer team does not shy away from the private sector. Pioneer team members recognized long ago that it can take years to find out whether a new idea will be widely adopted, and that with a relatively small budget, pioneer can only seed or boost innovation at an early stage. It requires investors with deeper pockets than pioneer and a willingness to persevere and cultivate demand for an innovation. These investors may be government agencies or other foundations—or perhaps other teams within the Robert Wood Johnson Foundation—but often the long-term hope of bringing a new technology to fruition is the private sector. Hence, the team's willingness to consider profit-motivated partners.

## —∿— Opening "Opportunity Spaces"

As the pioneer Portfolio has aged, the pattern of linking networks and forging creative relationships has become better understood as less a matter of serendipity and more one of deliberate cultivation and pursuit of certain areas. These are areas where the networks behind individual projects start to intersect and weave a bigger web of connections, cross-disciplinary communication, and creativity. For example, within a few years, experience with efforts like Project HealthDesign, the Rapid Learning project, and ARCHeS, among others, had begun to coalesce into a kind of intellectual ecosystem—something the team would later refer to as an "opportunity space." In recent years, the idea of an opportunity space—an area of innovative ferment and ripening opportunities for grantmaking—has come to demarcate any intellectual territory where pioneer team members collectively decide to spend more of their time in search of opportunities. The opportunity space that encompasses the data-based projects has come to be known as "real-world/real-time data," and the team has lately dedicated a portion of its resources for more concentrated exploration in that realm.

The cluster encompasses ideas for harvesting health information created in the course of daily life or business, and making it aggregated and stripped of identifying details, useful to researchers, health care providers, and policymakers. "We're on the verge of an explosion of data that we've never seen before," says Tarini, a former pioneer team director and now a senior program officer at the Foundation. "What do we do with it? How do we extract the signal from the noise? How does it get shared back with the people who are producing the data?"

Of the many possible answers to these questions, one may involve social media, in which people routinely share information on their day-to-day activities. Some of these online channels could offer a way to gather timely information on people's firsthand experiences with disease, treatment, and prevention. For example, an idea that germinated in pioneer's data-related opportunity space has been a relatively new partnership with a project called PatientsLikeMe, which *Forbes* described in 2013 as "producing some of the most compelling clinical data the health care industry has ever seen."[5]

Tarini tells the story of how the team met the three founders of PatientsLikeMe, James (Jamie) and Ben Heywood and Jeff Cole, MIT engineers in Cambridge, Massachusetts. Stephen Heywood, brother to James and Ben and longtime friend to Jeff, had spent years coping with Lou Gehrig's disease. Frustrated by the lack of practical information on the best ways to manage the illness and reduce suffering, in 2003 the engineers launched an online forum for patients with the disease. Thousands of people quickly found it extremely useful for exchanging information on treatments, nutrition, and other daily health experiences, and the number of subscribers soared. In 2005 and 2006, the founders expanded their forum to include other diseases. They also formalized their online efforts by forming a company that they believe "can transform the way patients manage their own conditions, change the way industry conducts research, and improve patient care."[6] Patients LikeMe currently has more than two hundred thousand users and continues to grow.

"PatientsLikeMe came to us," Tarini recalls. "They said, 'There are a lot of patient-reported outcome measurements out there. Some of them get used in research; some get used in clinical care. The ones that get used for research are really used to meet researchers' needs. The ones that get used in clinical care are used by providers to measure quality of care. There really aren't any patient-reported outcome measures that measure things that are really meaningful *to patients*. We want to build a platform . . . that a researcher, a clinician, an expert can use to build and validate outcome measures that patients report, and that are meaningful to patients.'"

The creators of PatientsLikeMe found pioneer largely because the team had by then become active in many of the business and intellectual networks where health-conscious innovators tend to gather. Tarini had first met Jamie Heywood, a founder of Patients-LikeMe, at a 2009 session of TEDMED, the health innovation forum. The two men then began what Tarini describes as "an episodic, running conversation for three years or so," before the discussions crystallized into a specific proposal. And the pioneer team was inclined to respond constructively to that proposal partly because its staff had also been in other conversations and meetings where real-world/real-time health data were front and center. The result of this intersection of networks was a $1.9 million Foundation grant in 2013 to PatientsLikeMe to create the Open Research Exchange, billed as "the world's first open-participation research platform for creating health outcome measurements."

Other opportunity spaces have taken shape in similar ways. One, called Games for Health, encompasses a suite of projects to explore the potential of video and computer gaming as a tool for improving health and health care. Another seeks ways of using behavioral economics both to improve the way health care is delivered and to solve persistent health problems. Might there be, for example, effective incentives for reducing the use of costly, but low-value, services in health care? If so, how should such incentives be employed? These webs of activity have emerged, connection by connection, from team members' early contacts and preliminary explorations of intriguing ideas—each leading to wider circles of thinkers and researchers probing related areas, and occasionally turning up candidates for pioneer support.

But before the formation of well-defined spaces and break-through opportunities, there first came months, often years, of what Paul Tarini calls "poking around": exploration, encounter, discovery, deliberation, and the occasional trips down blind alleys and around wrong turns. And yet it is precisely the latitude for these uncharted preliminary explorations, unrestricted by approved strategies and predefined objectives, that makes pioneer unusual. "The bulk of our work is through our networks—through the people we know and the people they know," Tarini says. "That's how we learn about ideas, that's how we learn about people, that's how we learn about developments."

## —∞— From Enabling to Breakthrough

In 2011 and 2012, the pioneer team set out to gather the lessons of their early years and to clarify the practices that have served them best. Among the principal findings of a strategic review completed in early 2012 was that, although identifying big breakthroughs may be the team's ultimate goal, it isn't the only important part of its work. "Poking around" and weaving networks have been more than just the means to an end. They have been valuable activities in themselves.

Before the strategic planning exercise, according to Brian Quinn, a former pioneer team leader and currently the Foundation's assistant vice president for research, evaluation, and learning "We were doing lots of different things, but we framed all of it as big breakthrough ideas that we were trying to support." The problem with that formulation is that not all of the ideas the team identified—not even all of its most promising and exciting ideas—would become disruptive innovations. It would take years, possibly decades, to know for sure which, if any, actually made a difference. In the meantime, however, the team will have been seeding and fertilizing important fields—fields whose intellectual energy and cross-disciplinary connections will have benefited from, and sometimes been partly shaped by, pioneer support.

"Despite the common metaphor of innovation as a 'lightning strike' of creative genius," the team wrote to the Foundation trustees in 2012, "transformative ideas rarely emerge out of nowhere. Systematically spurring innovation requires intentional processes and the careful nurturing of a set of conditions that make it possible to find, develop, and support new ideas in an ongoing way." The processes and conditions are themselves valuable products of smart philanthropy and should, therefore, be seen as key objectives, even if intermediate ones, for pioneer's work.

In its strategic review, the team came to define the earliest of these exploratory phases as "enabling processes," which "support general and open discovery to surface issues, approaches, and spaces to explore more deeply." These processes range from informal conversations to meetings with thinkers and innovators to hosting (or even just attending) conferences. They may also involve competitions like the one that eventually led the team to Project ECHO. There may be no pattern to the topics that surface in these early explorations, other than their relevance to health and health care. Over time, though,they have a tendency to draw attention, bit by bit, to more specific areas of opportunity.

Some of these will then become what the team calls "initial explorations," where team members investigate a particular topic. This may result in the team being able to develop a theory of change about how the topic should improve health. Ideas in this category have some common characteristics: they have at least some rough boundaries; there are identifiable networks of people thinking about or working on them or related projects; and there are promising leads to pursue and to probe. Of these kinds of ideas, the most fertile and the quickest to jell could eventually become opportunity spaces like the ones involving real-world data and games. The work in these spaces "will be time-limited and dictated by a theory of change about how investment can lead to breakthroughs."

Only at this point—when an idea has percolated through the early stages and become distilled into a concrete, testable proposition that can lead to significant change—does it qualify for treatment as a possible "breakthrough idea." According to the pioneer team's strategic plan, breakthrough ideas must have the potential to be genuinely transformational, that is, to improve health radically rather than incrementally. They must envision and address future conditions, not just current ones; be unconventional in the way they formulate and solve problems; and draw in approaches from multiple disciplines or sectors.

In that slow and time-consuming work, marked by meandering conversations and inchoate ideas, the most important discipline is receptivity. "Ideas may come from anywhere," former team leader Steve Downs notes, "including from fields that any one of us may know nothing about, or from combinations of fields that are unfamiliar or just plain weird." A willingness to consider ideas from unexpected, sometimes even uninvited, sources may be the feature that most distinguishes the pioneer team from its more strategically focused counterparts. Other Foundation teams do not accept unsolicited proposals; rather, they issue calls for proposals. At pioneer, spontaneous proposals have succeeded more than once.

One example of an idea whose odd juxtaposition of disciplines might arguably qualify as "just plain weird," but that eventually became an influential pioneer project, is Extending the Cure. A few years before the pioneer portfolio was created, Ramanan Laxminarayan, an economist with a master's degree in epidemiology, had submitted a proposal to the Foundation's public health team on ways of responding to the spread of infections that are resistant to today's antibiotics. Specifically, Laxminarayan was interested in the use of economic incentives similar to those applied to scarce natural resources, which aim both at conserving endangered assets (in this case, the effectiveness of antibiotics, which is depleted through overuse) and at encouraging the cultivation of new assets (here, the development of new and stronger antibiotics). His thesis was that if the right economic principles were applied, then laws, regulations, and professional practices could be devised to delay the march of antibiotic resistance and accelerate the creation of new drugs.

Although the problem was of general interest to the public health staff, the proposal's peculiar mix of disciplines and methods did not fit any of their strategic priorities. Knowing the odds against unsolicited proposals, Laxminarayan was neither surprised nor especially dispirited to be turned down. He was, however, intrigued to learn a year or two later that a new portfolio, called pioneer, was open to uninvited ideas. Better still, a member of the new team, Brian Quinn, had been grappling with policies on antibiotics earlier in his career and retained a keen interest in the subject.

So, Laxminarayan submitted again, this time to pioneer. Fearing that his emphasis on natural-resource economics might come across as a bit too eccentric, he toned down that element the second time around. Soon he was invited to meet with the whole team.

"I'd heard that the Foundation was interested in antibiotic resistance," he said recently, recalling that first meeting. "I thought what they wanted to hear would be everything to do with how drug resistance affected health care costs"—in other words, a traditional medical-economics approach. "Instead, their first question was, 'Where is all the stuff about thinking of this as a natural resource? That's what we're interested in.' I *never* thought they'd be interested in that. People think of resistance as a medical problem, and they get confused when you start talking about this whole other framework. But that is how I normally think about it."

Suddenly, Laxminarayan found himself engaged in more than a pitch; this was an actual conversation. Instead of the small planning grant he requested, he ended up with a six-figure research grant, and later a smaller grant to help promote the policy implications of his work.[7] The results included a long list of publications, including dozens of policy briefs and technical papers, anchored by a 170-page summary report, published in 2007, detailing the mounting dangers of antibiotic resistance, projecting the economic and human costs, and prescribing five interconnected policy solutions. Of these, three focused on reducing unnecessary demand for antibiotics and two on fueling production of new and more effective drugs.[8]

Extending the Cure is a project that members of the pioneer team regard with particular pride—in large part because it is typical of the kinds of initial explorations they consider a hallmark of the pioneer approach. But it's also because the project's effect on policy and public debate was noticeable and swift. Within months of the report from Extending the Cure, Senator Orrin Hatch cited it on the floor of the US Senate when he introduced a bill to address antimicrobial resistance. Some parts of Hatch's remarks echoed passages in the report. Thanks to support from the Foundation's Connect Project, which helps grantees present their ideas to members of Congress, Laxminarayan and his colleagues had met at least twice with members of the senator's staff in the weeks before his speech. "I don't know if they lifted the language from our report," Laxminarayan says, "or if they were even conscious of using that language. But the ideas obviously had an impact."

Senator Hatch's bill didn't pass; like many other important topics, it was overwhelmed by the financial crisis and national politics of 2008. But as if to demonstrate the staying power of the underlying idea, *Fast Company* spotlighted Extending the Cure more than five years later, in an article headlined "We Need to Treat Antibiotics as a Natural Resource." Still echoing the 2007 report, *Fast Company* described the solution to drug-resistant infections as "discouraging doctors from over-prescribing antibiotics, prodding pharmaceutical companies to release new drugs, and reducing overall demand to slow the evolution of new resistant strains."[9]

Admittedly, the story of Extending the Cure—arriving over the transom and nearly out of the blue—remains a relative rarity, even in the pioneer portfolio. Although unsolicited proposals get a hearing at pioneer ("We read them, every single one," former team director Quinn wrote on the team's blog), they still do not represent a big slice of the team's grantmaking.

## —⟋w— "Pitch Us"

In mid-2013, in a blog post titled "Pitch Us," the Foundation announced a wide-open invitation to new applicants: "On October 16, we're going to try a little experiment—a new way for you to share your ideas with us. We'll be hosting our first-ever pioneer Pitch Day in New York City. Over the course of two hours, eight teams will tell us their vision for how they want to change the world of health and health care—and how they plan to go about doing so. They'll be peppered with questions from me, my colleagues on the pioneer team, our grantees, and a few of our friends." Other than restricting each submission to no more than one thousand characters, Pitch Day had only one other rule: "Be original, be unconventional, be radical."[10]

The event drew more than five hundred submissions. From among eight finalists, a panel that included designers, investors, entrepreneurs, and journalists, as well as Foundation staff, picked three winners. One project involves new methods for cancer screening; another seeks better ways of harvesting medical knowledge online; the third uses social networks to improve patient safety in clinical settings. At the time this is written, the authors of all three submissions are working on fuller proposals for eventual funding.

Was this the first in a series of Pitch Days? "We're still evaluating the event (what worked well, what didn't work as well)," the pioneer website announced on October 22. "But the consensus seems to be that it's something we'll try again in the future. Stay tuned for more."

## —⟋w— Conclusion

Looking back on the first ten years, it seems fair to conclude that the creation of a pioneer portfolio has drawn in ideas and ways of thinking that might never have found their way into the Foundation otherwise. More than that, pioneer grants have helped to bring some of those new perspectives to a wider audience beyond the Foundation, and helped them influence thought, experimentation, and imagination on a broader scale. Some of these innovations may lead to genuinely disruptive change, though most are too young to say for sure. All of them, however, represent unfamiliar lines of work—some of them strikingly original, and a few that defy categorization.

Although the value of having a unit specifically charged with seeking out innovation may have been demonstrated, questions still arise about the place of an innovations unit within the organization. Pioneer was born primarily as a scouting expedition for ideas that could shape future programs at the Robert Wood Johnson Foundation. But it evolved into an idea lab exploring questions of health and health care more broadly, with only incidental influence on other Foundation teams went about their work. In the course of a strategic planning process throughout 2013, the senior leadership considered the role of pioneer within the Foundation. Should it be the research-and-development arm of the Foundation, looking for innovations that other teams can pick up? Should it be a quasi-independent unit whose role is that of identifying innovators and providing them with seed money to test their ideas until somebody with deeper pockets, such as a venture capitalist, comes along?

The answer—at least for the time being—is to maintain the pioneer team as the unit charged with finding and initially funding innovators, but to make its work more compatible with that of the rest of the Foundation. Pioneer is now the hub of efforts for the Foundation staff to learn from developments beyond the organization's Princeton, New Jersey, campus. It sponsors a regular speaker series that introduces innovators and iconoclasts—including speakers recommended by other teams—to the staff. This, along with guest bloggers and occasional panel discussions, is meant to contribute to what the team has called a "coffeehouse environment within the wider Foundation, where staff can learn, network, and connect ideas from an even wider variety of sources."

In the judgment of many people at the Robert Wood Johnson Foundation, including Lavizzo-Mourey, the willingness to cross boundaries and try out unfamiliar approaches is a vital institutional asset. "We have to learn deeply in certain content areas," she concludes. "But we also need to be constantly scanning the horizon, in this age when information is being created so quickly, and when there are so many fields relevant to improving health and health care for all Americans. When you look at the work of philanthropy, and what makes philanthropy able to do really great things, the key factor is understanding the fields that are out there, and how they are changing and intersecting and re-forming. Foundations need a mechanism for doing that."

## Notes

1. C. M. Christensen, *The Innovator's Dilemma* (New York: HarperBusiness, 2000); see particularly 54–63.
2. For a fuller description of Project ECHO, see S. Solovich, "Project ECHO: Bringing Specialists' Expertise to Underserved Rural Areas," in *To Improve Health and Health Care: The Robert Wood Johnson Anthology*, Volume XV, S. L. Isaacs and D. C. Colby, eds. (San Francisco: Jossey-Bass, 2012), 203–24.
3. See L. Wilson, "Advancing the Role of Rapid Learning in Mainstream Health Care," Robert Wood Johnson Foundation Program Results Progress Report, http://www.rwjf.org/en/research-publications/find-rwjf-research/ 2012/01/advancing-the-role-of-rapid-learning-in-mainstream-health-care.html.
4. See M. Nakashian, "Using Mathematical Modeling to Make Informed Choices on Health Care Alternatives," Robert Wood Johnson Foundation Program Results Report. http://www.rwjf.org/en/research-publications/ find-rwjf-research/2013/01/using-mathematical-modeling-to-make-informed-decisions-on-health.html.
5. B. Upbin, "PatientsLikeMe Is Building a Self-Learning Healthcare System," *Forbes*, March 1, 2013, http://www.forbes.com/sites/ bruceupbin/2013/03/01/building-a-self-learning-healthcare-system-paul-wicks-of-patientslikeme/.
6. From the PatientsLikeMe Web site, http://www.patientslikeme.com/ about.
7. See F. Feiden, "Extending the Cure: Policy Responses to the Challenges of Antibiotic Resistance," Robert Wood Johnson Foundation Program Results

Report, http://www.rwjf.org/en/research-publications/find-rwjf-research/2013/06/extending-the-cure--policy-responses-to-the-challenges-of-antibi.html.

8. R. Laxminarayan and A. Malani, "Extending the Cure: Policy Responses to the Growing Threat of Antibiotic Resistance," Washington, D.C.: Resources for the Future, 2007, http://www.extendingthecure.org/sites/default/files/ETC_FULL.pdf.

9. M. J. Coren, "We Need to Treat Antibiotics as a Natural Resource," *Fast Company*, August 5, 2013, http://www.fastcoexist.com/1682756/we-need-to-treat-antibiotics-as-a-natural-resource.

10. B. C. Quinn, "Pitch Us: The First-Ever Pioneer Pitch Day," *Pioneering Ideas* blog, August 13, 2013, http://www.rwjf.org/en/blogs/pioneering-ideas/2013/08/pitch_us_the_first-.html. 03chap_intro.doc

# CHAPTER 3

# OpenNotes

*Irene M. Wielawski*

## Introduction

Many health care experts see "consumer engagement" as a key to improving quality and lowering costs. But how to get people to be more actively involved in their own care has vexed these same experts for years.

Computers have unquestionably made things easier by enabling individuals, with a few clicks, to delve deeply into whatever health problem is bothering them; to learn about the advantages and risks of different treatments and medications; and, though they have not been widely used to date, to compare the cost and quality of different hospitals and physicians.

With the growth of electronic medical records, health care systems are now offering patients access to at least some of their medical records. But one kind of record has consistently remained off-limits: the doctor's own notes. Through a series of grants to Beth Israel Deaconess Medical Center generated by the pioneer team, the Foundation has been trying to change this. The program—called

OpenNotes—has been testing, in three different medical settings, the idea of patients having access to their physicians' notes.

In this chapter, Irene M. Wielawski examines the OpenNotes program in depth. Based on extensive interviews and visits to each of the sites, she concludes that the program has the potential to be a game changer (which is the goal of pioneer-generated programs). She cautions, however, that because OpenNotes appears to be popular and effective in primary care settings does not necessarily mean that it will be equally so in specialty settings—especially those, such as psychiatry and oncology, where the balance between openness and patient protection may have to be set differently.

Irene M. Wielawski, a frequent contributor to the *Anthology* series, is an independent writer and editor specializing in health care and policy topics. She has written extensively on socioeconomic issues in American medicine, particularly the difficulties faced by people who lack timely access to medical services because of financial, geographic, cultural, and other barriers.

Ellen Godfrey was crestfallen when her doctor of thirty years retired. She had invested a great deal in the relationship and the prospect of finding a replacement was daunting. How could she, at age seventy-two, establish the bond of trust that had taken so many years to build with her old doctor?

With trepidation, Godfrey phoned the doctor referral service at Beth Israel Deaconess Medical Center, the Boston hospital where she received most of her care. Presented with a roster of doctors who were accepting new patients, she chose the first name on the list. As it turned out, the doctor she selected was participating in a national experiment to give patients electronic access to their medical records—including the notes doctors write about them after an office visit or hospitalization.

Godfrey's previous doctor had vigorously opposed the idea of patients seeing their medical records, objecting even to sharing results of routine matters such as blood cholesterol tests. Godfrey had never quite understood why. A retired schoolteacher who still worked as a reading tutor, she liked knowing the details of things, including what was going on in her body. "I love being involved and that means staying healthy, so I want to understand my part in that."

So, when Godfrey received an e-mail offering her online access to her new doctor's notes, as well as to test results and prescriptions, she eagerly signed up. "I thought it was a great idea," she says. "You can't possibly remember everything a doctor tells you in an office visit. At the very least, I thought it would be a good way to document what was going on with my health, and remind me of medication instructions and things to do before the next visit."

Even so, Godfrey was a little nervous when she opened her new doctor's first note about her. "I was wondering what she thought of me," Godfrey recalls. "She's very young and I'm not—I was hoping that wouldn't get in the way of our understanding one another. The note was very long and detailed, and my first reaction was, 'Wow, this really took her a lot of time.' As I read it, I think it was a revelation to me that she had really listened because everything was there in the note, just exactly as we discussed it. I was so relieved. The accuracy of the note, and the ease with which we were able to discuss things, gave me confidence that I had found the right doctor."

—m—

Ellen Godfrey's experience with the national experiment known as OpenNotes illuminates the potential of including patients in clinical communications about their own diagnoses and treatments, thereby engaging them as partners in achieving and sustaining health. Proponents of such transparency say this is increasingly important for health care quality as patients shift from relying on a personal doctor to interacting with members of a clinical team, each of whom will have unique patient-care duties. Being able to read all these clinicians' notes could help patients better understand their medical conditions and reinforce the doctors' follow-up instructions. In return are potential benefits to the health care system.

Most of the illnesses that send people into the system today are chronic ones—cardiovascular disease, for example, or metabolic disorders such as diabetes—and they can be very expensive to treat. Although long-term studies are lacking, informed patients are widely believed to manage their conditions better, resulting in fewer crises and better treatment outcomes. At the very least, having access to their medical records would enable patients to monitor accuracy and fill in clinically relevant gaps in information.

Patients, moreover, are legally entitled to these medical records. The federal Health Insurance Portability and Accountability Act (HIPAA) of 1996 addressed a previously patchwork situation in which patients' rights to their records varied from state to state—and even where permitted, access was devilishly difficult and costly. HIPAA also set the stage for electronic sharing of these records with clinicians, health care organizations, insurance companies, researchers, and various government agencies.

But including patients in such streamlined point-and-click access has been slow—and intentionally limited. While some health care organizations have created electronic portals through which patients can schedule appointments, e-mail their health care providers, and see lab and other test results, doctors' narrative notes have remained largely off limits. The reluctance to share them with patients reflects a long-held professional view that these observational and interpretive findings are for clinicians' eyes only.

The OpenNotes experiment, which ran for twelve months in 2010 and 2011, challenged this insider culture, sparking debate about what constitutes appropriate communication with patients. In the end, most of the doctors who agreed to participate in the OpenNotes experiment were won over, and patients responded with striking enthusiasm. Several large health care systems have since added the option to their patient portals, fueling momentum for broader adoption and attracting new champions to help work out the bugs.

Like all true experiments, OpenNotes raised more questions than it could answer. Among them were concerns about the quality and communicative value of doctors' narrative notes. Simply put, they are all over the map in terms of clarity, accuracy, and completeness. If the idea behind sharing these records with patients is to engage them in sustaining health, how helpful is a file of poorly organized information replete with insider jargon and content gaps?

"We debate these questions endlessly," says Tom Delbanco, co-principal investigator of OpenNotes and professor of medicine at Harvard Medical School. "The beauty of what we're doing is that it's simple—and yet exceedingly complex at the same time. We're just at the Model T stage."

## —⚬— A Timely Idea

Comparing OpenNotes to the early days of the automobile is apt for the revolutionary change that OpenNotes' co-principal investigators—Delbanco and Jan Walker, a health services researcher and assistant professor of medicine at Harvard Medical School—set out to bring to the culture of medical practice. It was fitting, therefore, that after a nearly ten-year search for funding, Delbanco and Walker found a home for OpenNotes in the Robert Wood Johnson Foundation's pioneer portfolio, which specializes in novel ideas with the potential to be health system game changers.

On first review in early 2008, however, the pioneer program staff was unimpressed. "Our initial reaction was, 'What's the big deal here—just that you can get a record online?'" recalls Paul Tarini, an early reader of the grant application and, later, head of the pioneer team. "But as we talked about it, we realized that OpenNotes could potentially lead to an attitudinal shift in doctors towards their patients and improve the dialogue."

To refine the idea, Delbanco and Walker worked closely with Steve Downs, a member and, later, head of the pioneer team. Downs's background is in physics, which leads him to favor projects that are "simple and elegant" in design even as they tackle complex problems. He saw those elements in OpenNotes. Says Downs: "The knowledge that the note is being written not just for colleagues, but also for patients, we thought had the potential to change the way the doctors think about their patients."

In October 2008, the Foundation awarded Delbanco and Walker a fourteen-month planning grant of $118,000 to design a test of OpenNotes involving primary care doctors at three sites. The sites were selected to reflect the diversity of health care settings in the United States. In addition to Beth Israel Deaconess, which was the institutional recipient of the grant, the researchers recruited Geisinger Health System in rural Danville, Pennsylvania, and Harborview Medical Center, a public hospital in Seattle, Washington. In May 2009, the Foundation awarded Delbanco and Walker an additional $1,397,000 to implement OpenNotes at the test sites and evaluate the experience of participants. This was followed in 2011, 2012, and 2013 by awards of $647,000, $450,000, and $2,100,000, respectively, to expand adoption of OpenNotes at the experimental sites and develop tool kits for other institutions seeking to adopt the idea. OpenNotes also received financial support from the Drane Family Fund, the Florence and Richard Koplow Charitable Foundation, and the National Cancer Institute.

## —ᴧᴧ— To Share or Not to Share

In theory, transparency sounds like a wonderful thing. If we all had the same information, there would be a common basis on which to jointly identify problems, share ideas, and arrive at solutions.

But the degree to which anyone, in any realm, can truly lay it all on the table has long been a matter of debate. Politicians, scientists, merchants, soldiers, even families—all find reasons to hold back information or at least control the timing of its release both within and outside the group. Considered in this context, the fact that doctors selectively inform patients and make private judgments about when and how to convey certain details of diagnosis and prognosis should come as no surprise. Indeed, this has been the popularly accepted norm for centuries, and not just in the United States.

In part, this served historically to shield patients from how little medical science had to offer them in the face of infection, cancers, and most other ills. Keeping the truth from dying patients was seen as a kindness—as it sometimes still is. Even when the prognosis isn't so dire, the range of patients' personalities and competencies continues to influence what doctors say and how they say it—and contributes to their unease at the prospect of letting all of their patients automatically see raw, unmediated medical notes.

Patients' candor also ranges widely. Many are like Ellen Godfrey, eager to understand their conditions and to do the work necessary to sustain health. They are courteous and forthright in responding to questions about symptoms, medical history, and lifestyle that inform the diagnosis. But other patients lie about things like alcohol and drug abuse, diet, or how they became injured. They exaggerate or minimize symptoms and fail to follow medication or other instructions. Some demand prescriptions when none are warranted—and can become combative if they don't get their way.

Other patients are anxious and easily frightened, even by relatively minor findings. A few have psychiatric or neurological disorders that lead them to misinterpret or distort even basic communication. These patients are time consuming, difficult to manage, and sometimes frightening to have in the office. Why complicate matters by giving them access to blunt clinical communications containing their doctors' suspicions of, say, a cocaine habit, mental illness, or unsafe sex practice? Or, in the case of nervous patients, why heighten their distress with scary differential diagnoses—cancer? heart disease? brain tumor?—that pending tests could rule out?

Finally, not everyone wants to know the details of his or her illness or prognosis, or is in a condition to absorb the information. Compassion, sometimes demanded by family members, may lead to a softened or incomplete version of the truth. Indeed, it has long been considered part of the art of medicine for doctors to view the questions patients ask as indicators of how much information they want or feel prepared to handle.

Proponents of greater transparency in health care, however, say that medicine has lagged behind other professions, clinging to tradition and unwarranted paternalism even as patients turn to the Internet to research their diagnoses and treatment options. Old habits may die hard, but there's more to it than that. Transparency changes power dynamics, and that can be very disruptive in hierarchical cultures such as health care. The result has been little change, despite nearly five decades of discussion among medical leaders about the potential benefits of allowing patients to read and contribute to their medical records.

The OpenNotes research team knew this history well and, in pre-experiment surveys, corroborated these mixed feelings among doctors at the prospective test sites. Respondents wondered: Would patients be able to understand clinical notes since their main purpose is to communicate efficiently with other health care professionals? Did adding patients as readers mean the doctors would have to write their notes differently—or maybe dumb them down? Would the doctors subsequently be inundated with phone calls and e-mails from confused and possibly frightened patients? "Our doctors worried further about inappropriate reactions to what patients read," the research team reported in a 2010 article published in *Annals of Internal Medicine.* "They feared that some might become 'cardiac cripples' after reading descriptions of inconsequential arrhythmias, others might be devastated by an observation about mental illness, or speculations about cancer might trigger panic."[1]

Another complicating element was the clinicians' personalities. Doctors, too, vary in temperament and communicative skills. Through the surveys, the research team identified many areas of anxiety about sharing clinical notes with patients, ranging from the mundane—worries about awkward phrasing, poor spelling, and typos that might be off-putting to patients—to perceived violation of the medical profession's core principle: "First, do no harm." Clinical shorthand such as "SOB," referring to shortness of breath, could easily be misinterpreted, as could the use of "obese" to describe a patient who simply exceeds a recommended body/mass index. The standard professional phrasing "patient denies ..." as a means of systematically ruling out diagnostically relevant symptoms or behaviors might offend some readers. Collectively, the doctors were concerned that their notes might inadvertently cause "fear, frustration, guilt, anger, depression, confusion, or hopelessness," the researchers reported.[2]

Mostly, though, the doctors worried about extra demands on their time due to phone calls, letters, and e-mails from patients wanting to discuss or dispute the notes, and a consequent pressure to make notes less precise or complete in order to avoid patient blowback. "I was very uneasy," says Diane Brockmeyer, an internist with a specialty in domestic abuse cases who was among those surveyed. In addition to responsibility for about 750 patients at Beth Israel Deaconess, Brockmeyer wears a number of hats in the hospital's Healthcare Associates medical group, including directing quality initiatives in anticoagulation therapy. "I'm extremely busy, and although I'm a big fan of patient engagement, I just didn't want the hassle of dealing with a large amount of noise from patients that had no clinical benefit."

Surveys of patients also revealed misgivings. Some patients said they did not trust computers to deliver their medical records privately. Others shared the doctors' concerns about misunderstanding medical terminology, and a few said they would rather not know what their doctors wrote for fear of becoming anxious or reading critical comments. Several worried about the notes being a substitute communication that would lead their doctors to spend less time talking to them in person.

The surveys collected positive comments, too. Doctors perceived advantages in efficiency and clinical quality by, for example, giving patients lab test results in the same report as their doctors' interpretations and recommendations. Doctors also saw benefits for chronically ill patients and their families who might learn how to manage things better at home if they had notes to refer to for guidance. Patients, meanwhile, saw electronic access to their medical records as a "logical next step" in doctor-patient communication, and they were not daunted by the prospect of having to decipher medical terms.

"Many expected to search for explanations of technical language on the Internet," the researchers reported. "Some believed their doctor's notes would prove education simply by reminding them of what happened during the visit. They expected some notes to reassure them and to calm their fears; other notes might be 'truth tellers' and push them to face the reality of a health issue, such as obesity and mental illness, and perhaps break down defenses. Many liked the idea of sharing notes with family, friends, partners, and informal consultants, anticipating that this would help build a personal care system at home."[3]

## —⚕— Launching the Experiment

Collectively, 113 primary care doctors and 22,703 of their patients at Beth Israel Deaconess, Geisinger, and Harborview signed up to participate in a trial of OpenNotes. The dissimilarity of the test sites gave the experiment extra heft; not only were they located in different parts of the country, they also varied in institutional culture and resources available to support OpenNotes.

Boston's Beth Israel Deaconess is one of a cluster of internationally renowned academic medical centers affiliated with Harvard Medical School that attract patients, faculty, and students from around the globe. The hospital has been a national leader in deployment of new technology; its in-house electronic medical record system was the first in the United States to achieve the federal standard of "meaningful use." Beth Israel Deaconess was also an early adopter of the idea of Internet portals through which patients can make appointments and have access to their medical records—mostly test results until OpenNotes debuted.

Geisinger, an integrated health system with its own insurance plan, serves a mostly rural population in central Pennsylvania. It is the dominant health care provider in the region, with a tertiary-level hospital, community-based primary care practices, nursing homes, rehabilitation facilities, and home health agencies. Geisinger is often cited as a national model for team-based patient care and innovation in reducing health care costs without sacrificing quality. Like Beth Israel Deaconess, it has a widely used patient Internet portal.

Harborview is a public hospital caring primarily for poor and underserved patients, including prisoners, people with HIV and AIDS, victims of domestic violence, and substance abusers. Located at the top of what Seattle locals call "Pill Hill," the majestic 1930s-era Art Deco-style facility is one of the few public hospitals in the United States that runs in the black. This is partly due to its designation as a level 1 trauma center for the Pacific Northwest; the hospital also has several clinical areas of excellence that attract privately insured patients. Although county owned, Harborview is managed by the University of Washington, whose medical school uses the hospital as a site for teaching and research. Unlike Beth Israel Deaconess and Geisinger, Harborview and its network of outpatient clinics had no patient Internet portal before OpenNotes.

Each of these test sites had dedicated champions. At Beth Israel Deaconess, it was Delbanco and Walker. Although they are faculty of Harvard Medical School, both are based at the hospital. Walker has a nursing background and a Master's degree in business administration, and has long had a research interest in patients' experiences with health care. Delbanco, an internist, has been on the forefront of the movement to engage patients more actively in their care. Indeed, he was part of the research team in the 1990s that popularized the phrase "patient-centered care," now a fundamental principle of US health reform.

At Geisinger, the champion was Jonathan D. Darer, the health system's chief innovation officer. An internist with a Master's degree in public health, Darer had previously worked at Kaiser Permanente in Baltimore, where he had become interested in finding ways to leverage the existing health care infrastructure to achieve better population health. OpenNotes struck him as a useful tool in that pursuit, and he agreed to join Delbanco and Walker on the research team. "If you look at the success rates of people trying to quit smoking, it's about 3 percent overall," Darer says. "But if you can get the message to someone right after they've had a heart attack, you can get to 40 percent. So, timely communication can make a big difference both in the patient's response to medical advice and in their motivation. When the communication is also transparent, which is what OpenNotes promises, you can demonstrate to patients that you're working on their behalf—and that they should, too."

At Harborview, the OpenNotes champion was Joann G. Elmore, a professor of medicine at the University of Washington who at the time of the study was Harborview's chief of general internal medicine. Elmore brought to the research team a particular interest in improving the quality of doctors' notes. "There's too much abbreviation, jargon, mistyping, errors caused by cutting and pasting previous notes, and poor organization of information," she says. "OpenNotes is a useful teaching tool; our medical students need to learn to write clear, educational, and professional notes with the patient in mind as a reader."

In all three locations, the plan was to offer OpenNotes in outpatient primary care settings only, and to make participation by doctors and patients purely voluntary. To introduce the experiment and recruit doctors who would, in turn, make OpenNotes available to their patients, the researchers made presentations at medical staff meetings and also buttonholed individual doctors. Delbanco was particularly adept at the latter—with forty years on the Harvard faculty, he'd been a teacher to many doctors at Beth Israel Deaconess, and he used that leverage unabashedly. Darer was able to build on an already well-established Internet portal called MyGeisinger through which patients can schedule appointments, e-mail their doctors, and view lab test results. Some 225,000 people—40 percent of Geisinger's patients—have MyGeisinger accounts. Adding doctors' notes to the information they can access through this portal wasn't difficult, nor did it strike many patients as a big deal.

Elmore did not have the same technological advantages. Harborview had a homegrown electronic medical record system that solely served the communication needs of clinicians. To accommodate OpenNotes, the hospital's technical staff had to build one from scratch atop the existing system. This greatly limited the number of doctors and patients eligible for the experiment. But what Elmore did have was enthusiastic support for the OpenNotes concept from Harborview's executive director, Eileen Whalen. "I thought it was a no brainer," says Whalen. "We're a public hospital with a challenging patient population, some of whom have behavioral health issues, addictions, lives on the streets. So transparency is a big deal for us. We want to teach our patients to own their problems and be part of our wellness programs—and stay out of the hospital. OpenNotes fits right in with that."

The researchers also went out of their way to accommodate concerns raised by doctors and patients in the pre-experiment surveys and to underscore the voluntary nature of the OpenNotes experiment. At all three sites, doctors were assured that no extra writing would be required. They also were allowed to choose which of their patients would be invited to participate in the experiment. At Beth Israel Deaconess, the doctors were given the additional authority to withhold certain notes from patients. To address privacy concerns, participating patients received instruction in setting up password-protected Internet accounts through which they would receive their doctors' notes. Finally, all participants were told they could drop out of the experiment at any time.

## —ᴧᴧ— What Happened

Among other results, Diane Brockmeyer, the initially skeptical Beth Israel Deaconess internist, had a complete turnaround. "My expectations were completely off base," she says. "It turned out to be a lovely experience, and it was almost completely value-added. I've had dozens and dozens of experiences in which patients have said they were reminded to do something or were able to see how far they've come in the last year. It's been much less fuss than I anticipated."

Brockmeyer says she excluded a handful of patients because they were "overtly psychotic." At first, she also wrote her notes differently than she had when the expected readership was solely fellow clinicians. "I was conscious of using more partnering language in order to emphasize the shared decision-making," she says. But after the first twenty to thirty notes, she stopped trying so hard, although she believes her notes today are more patient-friendly. "In the beginning I was worried that there would be vocabulary and other comprehension issues, but that did not play out in my experience," she says. "I've had only two people call to correct information. Another patient expressed concern about personal information in a note and was very satisfied by my offer to put that note on monitoring (meaning it would not be routinely visible in the medical record)."

At the end of the experiment, 99 percent of participating patients wanted OpenNotes to continue, and none of the doctors who completed the experiment—105 out of 113, or 93 percent across the three test sites—chose to stop using OpenNotes. The data is stronger for doctors, almost all of whom filled out post-experiment surveys. Of 22,703 patients who initially signed up, 19,371, or 85 percent, completed the experiment. But only 13,654 actually got a note to open (the others did not have a doctor's visit during the trial period) and of these patients, 41 percent completed surveys.[4]

The data revealed a significant gap between doctors' and patients' perceptions of the value of open medical records. More than twice the percentage of patients as doctors "agreed" or "somewhat agreed" with post-experiment survey questions that timely access to clinical notes could help patients understand their medical problems, take better care of themselves, prepare for office visits, and comply with medication regimens.[5] Even more telling was the divergence in responses to questions about potential risks to patients of reading their medical records. At the end of the experiment, 13 percent of the OpenNotes doctors at Beth Israel Deaconess still thought the notes would be "more confusing than helpful" to patients. By contrast, only 2 percent of their participating patients thought so. Results at Harborview and Geisinger were similar, as was the gap between doctors and patients in their perceived risk of clinical notes' offending patients or making them anxious.[6]

These results tantalized the research team, who saw in the responses a need for more focused research on patients' wishes. "We know very little about how to actually engage patients," says Geisinger's Darer. "There are no outcomes data and everyone is trying to figure out what kind of information really matters and is helpful to patients. OpenNotes is a first step but there is so much more to do."

Interviews of patients who participated in OpenNotes illuminate the variety of ways in which they applied the knowledge gained from having access to their doctors' notes. Take, for example, the experience of Amanda Bengier: Bengier was already familiar with OpenNotes when she got her invitation to participate because she happens to work in Darer's innovation unit at Geisinger and had a hand in rolling out the experiment to clinicians. Still, she was amazed by how helpful doctors' written notes turned out to be in managing the health of her only child, Jack, six, who was born with spherocytosis, a hereditary form of anemia in which the body produces misshapen red blood cells that the spleen identifies as damaged and therefore works to destroy.

At the time of Jack's diagnosis, his serviceman father (the parents are now divorced) was deployed in Afghanistan. "I was pretty much on my own, and it took a good year or two for me to learn all the signs and symptoms to watch for—jaundice, pallor, fatigue, dark pee—that meant Jack was in trouble," says Bengier. "I'd take him to his doctor and try to absorb everything I needed to know to take care of him, but Jack would be running around, playing with the toys, and I'd be trying to manage him while also listening to the doctor and trying to memorize what he said."

OpenNotes brought order to this chaos, says Bengier. Reading doctors' notes on her home computer in the quiet of the evening, after she'd put Jack to bed, provided her with both ongoing education about the illness and a searchable record of her son's progress. She uses the notes like an online course, routinely looking up unfamiliar terms, even practicing their pronunciation in case someone asks her to explain a symptom. Bengier believes this has made her a better advocate for Jack, especially when she has to take him to the emergency room. "Spherocytosis is pretty rare—a lot of doctors have never heard of it," she says. "Because I'm up on the notes and the terminology, I'm able to let the emergency room people know why we're there and get Jack what he needs."

For Geisinger patient Robert Harter, sixty-two, a supervisor at the Wise potato chip factory in Berwick, Pennsylvania, OpenNotes is a practical solution to hearing problems that make it difficult for him to catch everything said in an office visit. Harter is deaf in one ear and has severe hearing loss in the other. "It helps to be able to read about what happened because when my doctor talks to me I might be catching only every third word," Harter says. "Also, I like seeing my test results before an appointment because it gives me something better to talk about when I go to see my doctor."

Eileen Hughes, fifty-two, of Jamaica Plain, Massachusetts, a community benefits program manager for Beth Israel Deaconess, has several chronic medical conditions, including type 1 diabetes and an autoimmune disorder, which require careful self-management. She uses OpenNotes for record keeping and to inform the dialogue during office visits, much as a clinician would. "When I arrive at my appointments, I've already reviewed my test results and notes from the last appointment so I can free up time to focus on more current issues with my doctor," she says. "I feel like my appointments are more satisfying as a result."

Timothy Kelley, fifty-six, of Auburn, Washington, came into the experiment already well educated about his primary illness, AIDS, having kept up on the latest science and treatments through Seattle's close-knit gay community. But keeping track of dosages and schedules for more than twenty prescription drugs is an ongoing challenge. "A lot of my medical appointments are related to drug side effects, and OpenNotes helps me monitor dosage changes, things like that," says Kelley, whose HIV infection dates back to 1994. "It also lets me correct errors in my medical record. For example, some of my meds weren't on the medication list and it's important for everyone to know what I'm taking. So we got that corrected."

Before OpenNotes, Kelley relied on a cheat sheet in his wallet. He would update it after every visit to Harborview's Madison Clinic, a dedicated HIV/AIDS facility that is part of a network of outpatient doctors' offices at the public hospital. But as Kelley developed new HIV-related conditions and other diagnoses—heart problems, allergies, type 2 diabetes—his neatly typed, single-spaced wallet list grew to three pages. OpenNotes makes it easier for him to review this complicated history and his doctor's advice; it also serves to reassure him that his views were "heard" during the office visit, even if his doctor didn't agree. "Sometimes, if I'm arguing about something I feel strongly about—like using herbal supplements on top of the medicines my doctor wants me to take—I don't always listen very well to the other point of view," says Kelley. "When I read the note later, sometimes I have to say, 'Yeah, I understand his point now and he's right.'"

Doctors who were interviewed also had a wide range of comments, both about their OpenNotes experience and about what may lie ahead as OpenNotes expands from primary care settings to outpatient specialty practices and clinics and, eventually, to the complex records of patients hospitalized for serious illness. The types of patients that these doctors see were often influential in their assessments.

Diane Brockmeyer, for example, the Beth Israel Deaconess internist who became an OpenNotes fan over the course of the experiment, has lingering concerns about privacy safeguards, particularly for patients who are victims of domestic violence and might come to further harm if private medical conversations are revealed. For this reason, Brockmeyer is grateful for the option at her hospital to put certain notes on "monitoring" so they're not easily accessible, even to medical personnel.

William E. Greenberg, chief of psychiatry at Beth Israel Deaconess, also has reservations, not so much for psychiatric outpatients as for those hospitalized with psychosis and other dangerous exacerbations of mental illness. "Our inpatient unit is a locked unit with a solid percent of patients who are there against their will," says Greenberg. "So these are not collaborative relationships of the sort one might have in an outpatient primary care setting. Yet other clinicians certainly need to know our patients' diagnoses and medications or if there's an eating disorder or some other influential condition. These are some of the discussions in our department about how to work with OpenNotes."

On the other hand, Geisinger's chief of rheumatology, Eric D. Newman, has not only embraced medical record transparency but has gone way beyond OpenNotes in using online communication tools with his patients. He credits his specialty for being unusually attuned to the benefits of doctor-patient collaboration, because virtually all of the patients seen in a rheumatology practice have incurable conditions that require a high degree of self-management and monitoring. Newman has his patients come early for appointments so they can sit at one of several computer terminals in the waiting area and type in answers to questions about what they have experienced since the last appointment. The responses hit Newman's computer screen before the patient walks through his door. "It lets us start the visit at thirty miles per hour," he says, and provides clinically important information that might not otherwise come up in an office visit.

Robert D. Harrington, medical director of Harborview's Madison HIV clinic, initially worried that OpenNotes would cause more harm than good due to the complexity of treatment of HIV-related illness, even in an outpatient setting. But he says he's only seen benefits in the small group of HIV patients handpicked to participate in the experiment (unlike at Beth Israel Deaconess and Geisinger where doctors excluded only a few of their patients, many were excluded at Harborview for such things as mental illness and substance abuse, as well as practical considerations such as whether they had access to a computer). Overall, according to Harrington, the patients who participated in OpenNotes seemed to have a better grasp of their medical problems, the reasoning behind various treatments, and the importance of compliance with medication regimens. "In HIV, adherence to treatment is the driver of good health," Harrington says, adding that public health is also served when HIV patients understand how the infection spreads and what they should do to prevent that.

Still, Harrington thinks the idea needs refining. "OpenNotes is a fire hose of information pouring into the patient," he says. "This, by itself, is not communication, although the information can facilitate communication and prompt important discussion that helps to engage patients in their care, which is very important. But I think we still have a way to go in understanding what kind of information patients actually find useful."

Harrington's colleague in the HIV clinic, Shireesha Dhanireddy, shares this view, wondering if there might be a middle ground between the paternalistic status quo and total transparency that takes into account the wide range of doctor-patient relationships. Many of these relationships are cut and dried—professional and cordial but not especially warm. But others are quite personal, for reasons that range from simply good chemistry to the emotional intimacy that develops when two people share a difficult journey. Dhanireddy recalls a favorite patient of long standing whom she enthusiastically recommended for OpenNotes, only to be dismayed by his reaction to reading her notes.

After the first note, the patient told her he did not want to read any more because the way they were written made him feel like just another sick person, rather than someone she cared about. "He felt completely objectified by my writing style which is very formal because my goal is to communicate with other clinicians as efficiently as possible," Dhanireddy says. "The note is not always reflective of the personal relationship."

—⁓—

## —⁓— Aftermath

How doctors express themselves in encounter notes was one of dozens of new areas of inquiry sparked by the OpenNotes experiment. Another was the inadequacy of current electronic medical records platforms, which tend to load billing information at the front end while burying doctors' notes, discharge summaries, medication instructions, and other information useful to clinicians and patients behind several screens. Still another concern was how to facilitate electronic access for people without computers. And throughout these post-experiment discussions rang the question: what do patients want?

Of the three OpenNotes test sites, Beth Israel Deaconess emerged as the most institutionally proactive. Indeed, executives there saw the 99 percent approval rating by patients in the experiment as a call to mandate medical staff participation.[7] By early 2014, all outpatient primary care and specialist departments at Beth Israel Deaconess are expected to offer OpenNotes to an estimated 225,000 adult patients eighteen and older; inpatient notes are projected to be available later in 2014.[8]

The speed of the rollout from a small primary care-based experiment to system-wide adoption reflects management's conviction that OpenNotes will give Beth Israel Deaconess a competitive edge in the crowded Boston hospital market. Behind the push is Kevin Tabb, the hospital's president and chief executive officer, who sees ramifications in OpenNotes beyond its popularity with patients. "OpenNotes is one step along the spectrum of transforming the relationship with patients into one of engagement and active participation," says Tabb. "For too long, hospitals have sat around waiting for very sick people to show up, thinking of themselves as being in the 'heads in beds' business. We looked, we diagnosed, we documented, and we didn't tell you anything. Today, we have to think differently about our patients—because we're in the health care business."

At Geisinger, the OpenNotes experiment was rapidly expanded in 2013 to all primary care practices, as well as to outpatient specialists—a total of some 550 doctors and advanced-practice nurses serving more than 120,000 patients. According to Jonathan Darer, another 300 clinical fellows and residents, as well as their supervising doctors, are expected to participate in 2014. But unlike Beth Israel Deaconess, Geisinger has chosen not to require participation. Rather, each medical department will be able to decide how and when to adopt OpenNotes, including whether to mandate it among department members or allow participation to be voluntary. The belief is that in the give-and-take within each clinical department, Geisinger's doctors will come up with ways to refine OpenNotes that might not surface were the medical staff simply ordered to participate. Darer and others point to the variability of concerns among specialists, especially those dealing with psychiatric or neurologically impaired patients, and the dearth of research data on patients' wishes. Studies of electronic communication tools in medical settings have focused almost exclusively on the information needs of clinicians and health care organizations.

Geisinger is also trying to improve the accuracy and utility of the notes. John B. Bulger, the health system's chief quality officer, has a growing list of expressions now banned from patient records due to their potential to cause error or misinterpretation. He has leaned on guidelines from The Joint Commission, an accreditation organization for hospitals, to compile it. For example, "MgSO4" and "MagSO4" as abbreviations for magnesium sulfate are barred because they can be dangerously misread as morphine sulfate. Everyone must now type out "magnesium sulfate." Also out are fractional dose measures rendered as, for example, ".5" rather than the newly mandated "0.5." This is because decimal points are easily overlooked on a shiny computer screen or handheld device, leading to ".5" being read as "5"—a tenfold increase in dosage.

Bulger is also working to address generational communication styles newly mucking up the medical record. Texting and social media shorthand, like "c u" for "see you," have lately cropped up as doctors speed-type their medical notes. This is not a great way to communicate with a broad-based patient population, says Bulger, nor with health care workers in the many settings in which a patient may be cared for: hospital, nursing facility, outpatient office, or home. "It used to be that the hospital staff rolled the patient out to the sidewalk for their ride home, thinking, 'That's it, I'm done,'" says Bulger. "But today we're dealing with a continuum of care, whether patients are in the hospital or being followed up by their own doctors. The notes have to provide reliable information for all of these providers. OpenNotes has the potential to increase this reliability because there's another set of eyes on the information and that's the person who really knows—the patient."

Finally, at Harborview, OpenNotes is being expanded from use by a select group of doctors and their patients to a standard offering of the outpatient adult medicine and ophthalmology departments. The hospital also plans to use OpenNotes in its residency training programs to teach new doctors better communication skills. Internist Jared Klein, a former chief resident and now a mentor to internal medicine trainees, is leading the initiative. "Residency is a key time for them to reflect on their interactions with patients, and to think about how to take the information they communicate face-to-face with patients and present it in a note that these same patients will read later," says Klein. "Right now, the notes are being driven by electronic templates primarily designed to elicit a billable minimum of services."

Klein believes this will be less of a problem if doctors learn early in their careers that patients, too, will be reading what they write. "I tell my trainees all the time: 60 percent of a doctor's job is communication, 30 percent is medical judgment, and 10 percent is medical knowledge. So skill in both verbal and written communication is key. I think OpenNotes can help me make that point."

Even as Beth Israel Deaconess, Geisinger, and Harborview work to refine and expand OpenNotes, the idea of giving patients electronic access to doctors' notes is spreading. At The University of Texas MD Anderson Cancer Center, 84 percent of active patients have electronic access to their full medical records, and the cancer center has looped in referring doctors as well.[9] A half million Cleveland Clinic patients are expected to be able to see doctors' notes by the end of 2013 via the clinic's online portal, MyChart.[10] And by early 2014, an estimated two million patients in the United States will be able to read their full medical records online. About a million of these are veterans using the Blue Button link on their My Health*e*Vet electronic portal. Launched by the US Department of Veterans Affairs in 2010, Blue Button gives patients electronic access to test results and medications so they can self-report medical histories, insurance status, and vital information such as weight and blood pressure. In January 2013, Blue Button opened patients' entire medical records, including doctors' notes.[11]

## —⚬— Conclusion

So convinced was Timothy Kelley of the benefits of reading his doctors' comments that he set out to gather his medical records going back to when he was first diagnosed with HIV in 1994: "I wanted to see what I was doing when my health deteriorated and what I was doing when I was getting better so I could continue those things and keep my health."

Kelley had to request paper copies, because OpenNotes provided computer access only to records from 2010, when the experiment began. This is where Kelley's legal right to these records foundered amid the small print of HIPAA that permits health care providers to charge a fee for photocopying. At Harborview, the rate is currently twenty-six cents a page. "I was only able to get the records back to 2006 before I had to stop due to finances," says Kelley, who lives on Social Security disability stipends. "It cost me over $150 so I have to wait until I save some money to go back further."

It turns out that Harborview's rate is a bargain. Although federal law requires health care organizations to provide patients with their medical records, state laws define the process of obtaining them, including setting copying fees. These fees vary from state to state. Colorado, for example, allows fees up to $14 for the first 10 pages, 50 cents a page for pages 11 to 40, and 33 cents a page for the rest.[12] Florida permits fees of up to $1 a page for the first 25 pages and 25 cents per page after that.[13] New York allows charges of up to 75 cents per page.[14]

The culture that OpenNotes sought to change is manifest in these laws and business practices which, besides creating cost barriers for patients like Kelley, dictate an elaborate process for them to follow, including: written requests on approved forms, separate applications for each record, notarized signatures in some jurisdictions, and waiting periods of up to thirty days. As if to underscore the double standard, many states explicitly exempt doctors and health care organizations from these fees and process requirements when they request patient records. In the context of current thinking about the importance of patients working collaboratively with health care personnel, such fees and procedural hoops are at best counterproductive. They call to mind the discouraging toll-free customer phone services that keep people on hold for so long that they simply hang up. "We have to find a better way of connecting the many parts of our health care life," says Risa Lavizzo-Mourey, president and CEO of the Robert Wood Johnson Foundation, who sees OpenNotes as a tool to that end. "Part of that is redesigning the health care delivery system in a way that puts the patient in the center and population health as a priority."

With regard to the inadequacies of current electronic medical record design, in which billing codes and other non-clinical data obscure the display of doctors' notes and other information useful to patients, there is nothing preventing health care organizations and vendors from collaborating on improvements. These electronic platforms began as billing systems with the medical information included as backup documentation for claims. It seems a simple thing to pursue redesigns on behalf of patients and clinicians, especially given the billions of dollars in federal subsidies for health care providers to encourage meaningful use. In fact, OpenNotes leaders Delbanco and Walker have discussed the issue with a leading electronic medical record vendor, and Geisinger is pursuing an in-house fix by adapting its existing electronic medical record platform to support OpenNotes.

Less obvious is how to deliver medical records in a way that supports *patients'* meaningful use. The questions raised by Harborview's Harrington and others about the value of spraying a "fire hose" of technical information at patients are not so easily answered (see the samples of medical record notes reprinted in the appendix). And new questions will surely arise as OpenNotes moves from the primary care setting into specialties that treat patients with more medically complex problems, including cognitive and psychiatric disorders.

Such discussions are perhaps the richest legacy of the OpenNotes experiment—an idea whose impact is likely to extend well beyond what even those who conceived of the project could have envisioned. Among doctors and patients who field-tested OpenNotes, the tool has clearly helped to break down the us-versus-them mentality that historically colored their relationship. The challenge for those moving swiftly to replicate and expand OpenNotes is to keep patients in the research loop.

Geisinger's Darer notes the dearth of information on patients' wishes. How they use OpenNotes and deploy its benefits in daily life are critically important questions to answer if the health care system is to realize the theoretical promise of patient engagement: better population health at lower cost.

## —⟞⟞— APPENDIX

### *Sample Medical Records*

## (The following are actual records redacted to protect the privacy of the patients.)

Sample Note # 1

```
Note Date:
Signed by .            , MD on           at      pm Affiliation:

VS: Wt. 160 lbs BMI 22.3 Kg/m2 P 56 BP 144/90
--------------- ---------------- ---------------- ----------------
Active Medication list as of .       :

Medications - Prescription
AMLODIPINE - 10 mg Tablet - 1 Tablet(s) by mouth once a day
HYDROCHLOROTHIAZIDE - 25 mg Tablet - 1 Tablet(s) by mouth once a
day
LISINOPRIL - 30 mg Tablet - 1 Tablet(s) by mouth once a day
METOPROLOL TARTRATE [LOPRESSOR] - 100 mg Tablet - 1 Tablet(s) by
mouth twice a day

Medications - OTC
ASPIRIN [ASPIRIN CHILDRENS] - 81 mg Tablet, Chewable - 1
Tablet(s) by mouth daily
--------------- ---------------- ---------------- ----------------
HISTORY OF PRESENT ILLNESS:        is here after an overnight
admission to              hospital, where he was seen with,
syncope, hypokalemia and paroxysmal atrial fibrillation. He has
subsequently been seen there by a cardiologist who called me and
wondered if he might have amyloid, without realizing that he had
a long history of hypertension.

He left there on new dosages of medicines, but the same
medicines, and he will call me later today with the exact dosages
of what he is taking.  He does not have them with him.  While at
the hospital, he had numerous evaluations, but he was felt safe
to leave, and is tired of being seen out there and wants to
return to care here.  I am delighted to have him back.

He feels fine now.  He does not get the same monitoring at work
that he used to because his nurse left, but right now he feels
pretty much back to normal.  He is back to work.

They told him apparently that he was on "too much medicine," and
I assume they meant by that the hydrochlorothiazide, given his
hypokalemia, but he is not sure which medicines have been
changed.

Of note is the fact that his stress test here in March was
basically fine.  He has not had an x-ray here in seven years and
I will repeat that today (unchanged and not particularly
remarkable).  We will also take a look at his cardiogram and of
course check his electrolytes (K+ on the low side, bicarbonate on
the high side).
```

```
PHYSICAL EXAMINATION:
GENERAL:  On evaluation today, he looks well.
VITAL SIGNS:  His blood pressure is 144/88 by me, sitting, and
the same supine.  His pulse is 60 and entirely regular over 2
minutes.  His weight is stable.
LUNGS:  Clear.
HEART:  I do not hear adventitious cardiac sounds.  There is no
sign of cardiac decompensation.
ABDOMEN:  His liver is not enlarged.
NECK:  His veins are not distended.
EXTREMITIES:  His ankles are fine.

ASSESSMENT AND PLAN:  It sounds to me as if much of this was
induced by hyperkalemia, and we shall have to indeed check that
out over time and likely change his regimen.  I have urged him
for now to eat lots of bananas, and drink lots of orange juice
```

## Sample Note #2

### Infectious Disease - Inpt Record

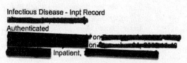

\* Final Report \*

Result Type:      Infectious Disease - Inpt Record
Service Date:
Result Status:    Authenticated
Performed By:                              on
Verified By:                              on
Encounter info:               Inpatient,

**\* Final Report \***

### Infectious Disease Consult Follow-up Note

### Hospital Day: 26

### ID & Chief Concern/Problem *(required for all billing levels)*

year old man with A3 HIV and polysubstance abuse who presents with multiple complications
of cocaine overdose, multi-system organ failure and cavitary PNA.

### Interval History/Major Events *(past 24 hours)*

Yesterday, pt self-extubated and required prompt re-intubation.  He continues on minimal
settings on the vent.  He is euvolemic and continues on intermittent HD.  He has spiked high
fever to >40oC on 12/2, but has been afebrile since.  He had CT imaging of the C/A/P that
showed similar cavitary lesions of lung, liver, spleen similar to prior CT chest and also what
appeared radiographically to be necrosis in the psoas.  We are currently treating for
stenotrophomonas, citrobacter and MRSA in the lungs as well as empirically for fungemia.

Antimicrobials:
Vanco 11/11-current
Meropenem 11/11-12; 11/29-current
Moxifloxacin 11/22-current
Flucon 11/27-current
Acyclovir 11/22-current
Pip/tazo: 11/17-11/22
Ceftriaxone 11/12-11/17
Outpt: TDF/FTC/Fosamprenavir/r

Infectious Disease - Inpt Record

* Final Report *

**Review of Systems** [x] Unable to Obtain due to Patient Condition
CONSTITUTIONAL [ ] Negative _ EYES [ ] Negative _ ENMT [ ] Negative _
CARDIOVASCULAR [ ] Negative _ RESPIRATORY [ ] Negative _ GI [ ] Negative _
GENITOURINARY [ ] Negative _ NEURO [ ] Negative _ MUSCULOSKELETAL [ ]
Negative _
SKIN [ ] Negative _ ENDOCRINE [ ] Negative _ ALLERGY/IMMUNOLOGY [ ] Negative

HEME/LYMPH [ ] Negative _ PSYCHIATRIC [ ] Negative _

**Allergies**
NKA

**Scheduled Medications**
Acyclovir susp (conc 40mg/mL)  Dose: 200 mg = 5 mL Feeding Tube  QDay
Calcium carb 1250mg(elem 500mg)/5mL susp  Dose: 1,250 mg = 5 mL Feeding Tube  Q8
Hours
Chlorhexidine gluconate 2% topical cloth  Dose: 1 application Topical  QHS
CONCENTRATE IV MEDS IN NORMAL SALINE  Dose: 1 each MISC  QDay
Heparin 5,000units/mL inj  Dose: 5,000 units = 1 mL Subcutaneous  Q8 Hours
Lansoprazole 30mg soluble tab  Dose: 30 mg = 1 tab Feeding Tube  QDay
Lidocaine/Diphenhydramine/Al-Mg hydroxid  Dose: 15 mL PO  BID
Meropenem  Dose: 1 g IVPB  Q24 Hours
Moxifloxacin/0.8% NaCl  Dose: 400 mg = 250 mL IVPB  Q24 Hours
Phenytoin 300mg/12mL susp  Dose: 300 mg = 12 mL Feeding Tube  Q12 Hours
Sedation Vacation  Dose: 1 each MISC  QAM
Sodium chloride 0.9% inj 10mL (syringe)  Dose: 10 mL IV Push  Q8 Hours
Vitamin multiple, with mineral 15mL soln  Dose: 15 mL Feeding Tube  QOther Day

**Infusions**
Dextrose 5% in Water 850 mL + Sodium bicarbonate 150 mEq  Dose: 850 mL IV Infusion
Fentanyl 5,000 mcg + Diluent 100 mL  Dose: 100 mL IV Infusion
Lorazepam 40 mg + Dextrose 5% in Water 20 mL  Dose: 20 mL IV Infusion
Sodium Chloride 0.9% 1,000 mL  Dose: 1,000 mL IV Infusion

**PRN Medications** *(Please, see the medication profile)*

## Infectious Disease - Inpt Record

\* Final Report \*

### Vitals *(Most recent and 24 hour range.)*

| Date | | Result | Last | MIN | - MAX |
|------|------|--------|------|-----|-------|
| 12/ | 08:05 | Temp C: | 37.4 | 36.7 | - 37.4 |
| 12/ | 11:01 | HR: | 104 | 100 | - 110 |
| 12/ | 11:01 | RR: | 17 | 16 | - 42 |
| 12/ | 11:01 | SBP Non-Inv: | 97 | 87 | - 117 |
| 12/ | 11:01 | DBP Non-Inv: | 59 | 52 | - 75 |
| 12/ | 11:01 | MAP Non-Inv: | 70 | 61 | - 86 |

### Neurophysiology Data *(Most recent, lowest and highest for 24 hour range)*

| Date | | Result | Last | MIN | - MAX |
|------|------|--------|------|-----|-------|
| 12/ | 08:09 | GCS Total | 10 | 10 | - 14 |

### I&O Data
Height: 173.0 (cm) 5' 8" (ft / in) (11/     )
Admit Wt: 79.30 (kg) 174 (lbs) (11/     )
Last Daily Wt: 68.4 (kg) 150 (lbs) (12/    05:00)
Previous Daily Wt: 68.7 (kg) 151 (lbs) (12/    04:00)

(24 Hour IO Total = from 06:00 the prior day to 05:59 listed day)

| Result | 12/ | 12/ | 12/ | 12/ | 12/ | Total |
|--------|-----|-----|-----|-----|-----|-------|
| Intake Total (0600) | 1817 | 1931 | 1742 | 1721 | 431 | 7642 |
| Output Total (0600) | 0 | 837 | 45 | 750 | 320 | 1952 |
| Net I&O Total (0600) | 1817 | 1094 | 1697 | 971 | 111 | 5690 |
| Daily weight | 67.6 | 69 | 68.7 | 68.4 | | N/A |

### Respiratory Data *(Most recent and 24 hour range.)*
| Date | 12/    08:40 |
|------|------|
| Ventilator Mode: | AMV |
| O2 Sat: | 100 |
| O2 Percent Administered: | 30 |
| O2 Delivery Device: | Ventilator |

### PHYSICAL EXAM
Gen: intubated/sedated
Neuro: lightly sedated, responsive to voice, follows commands in spanish

## Infectious Disease - Inpt Record

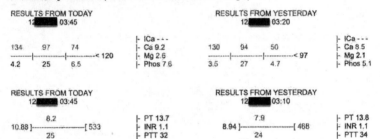

* Final Report *

HEENT: PERRL, anicteric, purulent ulcer on the right upper lip.
CV: RRR no murmer, no edema
Pulm: course mechanical BS anterolaterally
GI: NABS, soft, NT
Skin: opened bullae over patella b/l are healing

### Laboratory Studies *(Most recent results in 24 hour range.)*

RESULTS FROM TODAY
12 ▮ 03:45

```
                          |- ICa - - -
134    97     74          |- Ca 9.2
----------|----------|----------< 120   |- Mg 2.6
4.2    25     6.5         |- Phos 7.6
```

RESULTS FROM YESTERDAY
12 ▮ 03:20

```
                          |- ICa - - -
130    94     50          |- Ca 8.5
----------|----------|----------< 97   |- Mg 2.1
3.5    27     4.7         |- Phos 5.1
```

RESULTS FROM TODAY
12 ▮ 03:45

```
        8.2               |- PT 13.7
10.88 }----------------[ 533   |- INR 1.1
        25                |- PTT 32
```

RESULTS FROM YESTERDAY
12 ▮ 03:10

```
        7.9               |- PT 13.8
8.94 }----------------[ 468   |- INR 1.1
        24                |- PTT 34
```

### Last 6 Hematocrits in Preceding 24 Hours
*(NOTE: Comments/notes for Labs are viewable on Flowsheet)*

```
12 ▮      12 ▮
03:45     03:10
 25        24
```

### ABG Results
*(NOTE: Comments/notes for Labs are viewable on Flowsheet)*
7.40 / 40 / 131 / 24 / Calculated O2 SAT not reported. / 40 / Information not provided

### Other Results
--

### Radiological Studies

CT Chest/Abd/Pelv (12/2)

Printed by: ▮
Printed on: ▮

Infectious Disease - Inpt Record

* Final Report *

IMPRESSION:
1.Fluid collections within the lung parenchyma are suspicious
for abscesses. Surrounding consolidation is compatible with
pneumonia, with small bilateral parapneumonic effusions.
2.Bilateral psoas muscle enlargement with areas of necrosis is
likely rhabdomyolysis in patient with this clinical diagnosis.
Alternatively it could represent hemorrhage or infection.
3. Peripheral irregular hypodensities in segment 7 of the liver
again most likely are small infarcts.  These are not
significantly changed since prior exam.
4.Wedge-shaped low-density regions in the spleen are not
significantly changed since prior exam again likely reflect
infarcts.

## Microbiology

11/30: BAL- LLL GPCs & GNRs: see cultures 11/28 (>30,000col/mL of non-LF GNRs)
11/28: ET sputum: 2+ stenotrophomonas, 2+ MRSA
11/24: Pleural fluid: NGTD
11/24 & 26: ETT: 2+ stenotrophomonas, 2+ citrobacter
11/22: penile: pending HSV. negative GC/CT, RPR
11/20: lip: HSV-1
11/19: ETT: 2+ stenotrophomonas, 2+ citrobacter
11/15 (BAL): MSSA, Citrobacter #1,2, neg: flu, viral, AFB, aspergillosis
11/14 arthrocentesis (b/l knees): NGTD
11/12 NP swab: Neg: flu
11/11 Sputum (ET): 4+ citrobacter braakii #1, 4+ S. pneumo, 3+ MSSA, 3+ C. braakii #2
11/10-11 Blood (periph & HD cath): S. pneumo
11/8  Sputum (ET): 3+ H. influenazae, 1+ MSSA, 3+ S. pneumo, 2+ yeast

## Problems / Assessment / Plan

 year old man with A3 HIV and polysubstance abuse who presents with multiple complications
of cocaine overdose, multi-system organ failure and cavitary PNA. Pt seems to be making very
mild clinical improvement based on the afebrile since almost 48 hours.  However, the psoas
abscesses are concerning for necrosis vs. infection, especially in the setting of initial S. pneumo
bacteremia and we would recommend sampling these to determine sterility.  Also, the
stenotrophomonas should probably be covered by a second active agent and micro plate rounds
today determined that the MICs for moxifloxacin are borderline; the lab will be running
sensitivities on the stenotrophomonas from the BAL on 11/30.  Active agents against his bug are

Infectious Disease - Inpt Record

* Final Report *

TMP-SMX and minocycline with TMP-SMX having better activity.

## Recommendations
- consider IR sampling of psoas fluid collection
- agree with current ABx regimen
- recommend adding TMP-SMX (tmp componenet 7.5mg/kg) IV qday

Thank you for the opportunity to participate in the patient's care. We will follow closely with you. Please call with any questions.

**Attending Statement:**
I did not see the patient, but have reviewed the findings above.

Signature Line
Electronically Reviewed/Signed On: ▮▮▮ at 16:21

Resident, Department of Medicine

Electronically Co-Signed On: ▮▮▮ at 16:43

Attending, ▮▮ Dept. of Medicine
Division of Allergy and Infectious Diseases, ▮▮▮

Printed by:
Printed on:

Infectious Disease - Inpt Record ▮▮▮▮▮▮▮▮▮▮▮▮▮▮▮

* Final Report *

JDG
DD: ▮▮▮▮▮▮

Sample Note #3

## * Final Report *

### Surgery Admit/Consult Note

**Dept Surgery: Initial Hospital** [_] **Admission** [X] **Consult**

**Date:** ████████    **Time:** 1500    **Pt Location:** ED

Consult requested by:ED    Reason:concern for bowel obstruction
Consult request template viewed in requesting service progress note: [_]

**Completed by:** [X] Resident [_] Fellow [_] Attending
**Surgery Attending:** _
**Service:** [_] 1 [_] 2 [_] Thor [_] Vasc [X] A [_] B [_] S

**ID/CC:**
fever, abdominal pain

### HPI:

The pt. is a XX y/o gentleman with a PMHx significant for Crohn's disease complicated by entero-enteric fistula, chronic abdominal pain for a few months resulting in decreased PO intake and weight loss of 20 pounds over the last several months. The pt was seen in surgery clinic (Dr. XXXX) on ████████nd CT revealed significant inflammation of the distal ileum, ileocecal valve and cecum. The pt was scheduled for surgery in early August for removal of the effected areas.

Today the pt present with a few day history of abdominal pain, distention, with decreased stool and flatus. Pt reports some fevers. Positive bilious vomiting prior to presentation to the ER. He reports that his abdomen did not feel distended to him.

### ROS:

[_] Unable to obtain history due to patient intubation, sedation, other incapacity, unable to obtain from alt source.

Const: [_] negative  Comments:as in HPI

Eyes:  [X] negative  Comments: _

ENMT: [X] negative  Comments: _

CV:    [X] negative   Comments: _

Resp:  [X] negative  Comments: _

GI:    [_] negative  Comments: _

GU:    [_] negative  Comments: as in HPI

MSK:   [x] negative  Comments: _

Skin:  [x] negative  Comments: _

Psych: [x] negative  Comments: _

Endo:  [x] negative  Comments: _

Lymph: [x] negative   Comments: _

Allergy: [x] negative   Comments: _

**Past, Family, Social History:**


PAST MEDICAL HISTORY:
1.  As in HPI.
2.  GERD.

PAST SURGICAL HISTORY:
Wisdom teeth removal.

ALLERGIES:
NO KNOWN DRUG ALLERGIES.  HOWEVER, HE STATES THAT MORPHINE GIVES
HIM HALLUCINATIONS.

CURRENT MEDICATIONS:
1.  Humira 40-mL injection every 2 weeks.
2.  Hydrocodone 5/325 1 to 2 pills q4-6h as needed for pain.
3.  Ciprofloxacin 500 mg PO twice daily.
4.  Metronidazole 250 mg PO twice daily. )

SOCIAL HISTORY:
The patient lives in XXX with his XXX and X children.  He is a
manager at XXXX.  He denies drug, tobacco, or alcohol use.

FAMILY HISTORY:
1.  The patient states that he has a family history first-line
brother 34 Crohn disease.
2.  Father died of MI at age ▆▆.


**Exam:**


**VITAL SIGNS:** Temp: 36   BP: 121/70   Pulse: 96   Resp: 20   Weight: _kg   SaO2: 98% on RA
        Vital Sign Assessment                [_] Normal [x] other: borderline tachycardia

**GENERAL:** _
**HENT:**        [_] perrl, eomi, oropharynx clear [_] icterus [_] other: _
**HEAD/NECK:**  [_] supple, no thyromegaly, no bruits  [_] other: _
**LYMPH:**       [_] no lymphadenopathy
                [_] lymphadenopathy: [_] neck [_] supraclavicular [_] axilla [_]groin [_] other: _
**CVS:**         [X] rrr, s1s2, no m/r/g [_] other: _
  Extremities: [_] no c/c/e  [_] edema B 1+/2+/3+/4+  [_] other: _
  Pulses          <u>Right</u>          <u>Left</u>          <u>Right</u>          <u>Left</u>
                  Fem _          Fem _          Pop _          Pop _
                  Dp _           Dp _           Pt _           Pt _

Carotid: _
Other CVS: _

**RESP:**     [] CTA bilaterally  [_] crackles  [_] expiratory wheezes _  [_] other: _
**SKIN:**     [_] warm, dry, no jaundice/sig lesions/rashes  [_] jaundiced  [_] other: _
**BREAST:**  [_] normal  [_] other: _
**GI:**       decreased BS, soft, +TTP in supra-pubic region and RLQ. No round tenderness, no gaurding.
        Hernia: [_] no hernias  [_] ventral/inguinal/femoral [_] incarcerated  [_] other: _

**KEY PHYSICAL EXAM FINDINGS:** TTP in RLQ and supr-pubic regions

**Labs:**
WBC 26
Alb 3.2
UA: WNL's

**Studies/Records Reviewed:**
Acute abd series: dilated loops of small bowel with air/fluid levels, no free air under diaphragm

CT abd/pelvis:  Small bowel is diffusely distended up to the terminal ileum, where
there is short segment of diffuse circumferential wall thickening,
lumenal narrowing, and mesenteric fat stranding. The colon is unremarkable.  No abscess or fistula is identified.

**Resident Assessment & Plan:**
The pt. is a XX y/o gentleman with a PMHx significant for Crohn's disease complicated by entero-enteric fistula, chronic abdominal pain for a few months resulting in decreased PO intake and weight loss of 20 pounds over the last several months. Pt. now with fever, vomiting and elevated WBC. Abd series suggestive of small bowel obstruction, CT abd/pelvis reveals no identifiable fluid collections, but an area of thickened bowel wall in the ternimal ileum. The pt has a bowel obstruction secondary to a Crohn's flare and known terminal ileal stricture disease scheduled for elective surgery by Dr. XXXX in late August.
-recommendations:
-admit to medicine
-obtain GI consult for medical management of Crohn's flare
-cont. NPO, NG-tube, bowel rest
-IV antibiotics
-TPN
-Surgery will continue to follow and if pt worsens or does not improve will consider taking the pt to the OR for surgical intervention, however ideally the pt. will improve so that the procedure may be down electively.

**Resident pager Number:**
XXX-XXXX


**ATTENDING STATEMENT:**
I personally saw and evaluated the patient. I discussed the patient with Dr. XXXX. I agree with the findings and plan as documented in his/her note.
Whether this patient needs surgery in the near future or electively in Aug as planned, it is very important that he doesn't lose any more nutritional decline.   Strongly recommend TPN asap.

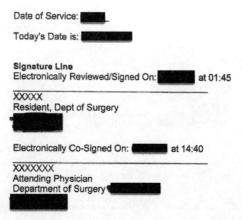

Date of Service: ▆▆▆▆

Today's Date is: ▆▆▆▆▆

**Signature Line**
Electronically Reviewed/Signed On: ▆▆▆▆ at 01:45

_____

XXXXX
Resident, Dept of Surgery
▆▆▆▆

Electronically Co-Signed On: ▆▆▆▆ at 14:40

_____

XXXXXXX
Attending Physician
Department of Surgery ▆▆▆▆
▆▆▆▆▆

AGH
DD: ▆▆▆▆

Sample Note #4

## Breast Care - Outpt Record

* Preliminary Report *

Result Type:          Breast Care - Outpt Record
Service Date:
Result Status:        Transcribed
Result Title:
Performed By:                              on
Encounter Info:                  Outpatient,

### * Preliminary Report *

ROOSEVELT BREAST CLINIC NOTE

IDENTIFICATION
█████████ is a ██ year-old Hispanic female who is referred this date by ███████████ for evaluation in regard to a left breast abscess.

CURRENT BREAST PROBLEM
The patient apparently developed swelling, erythema and a raised area in the left breast approximately 3 months ago. She was subsequently seen and evaluated and treated with clindamycin, which improved her pain and swelling somewhat. However, the pain, erythema and swelling subsequently returned. She was then seen again in December in a local ER and treated with vancomycin. She developed a rash on vancomycin and this was discontinued. She was then seen in the █████████ on January 11, ███,and started on Keflex 500 mg 4 times a day. Her symptoms did not improve and she was subsequently seen in the █████████ on January 11, ███ At that time, she was noted to have diffuse erythema in the area of fluctuance at the 7 o'clock position in the left breast. An ultrasound was completed and revealed a superficial abscess at the 7 o'clock position measuring 4 x 8 x 2.5 x 3.8 cm. This was noted to be immediately inferior and medial to the nipple and extending deeply into the breast in the medial and superior directions.

The decision was made to proceed with I&D, which was completed on January 11, ███ The patient was then discharged on Bactrim DS and instructed to take 2 tabs twice daily. She was also provided with oxycodone, Tylenol and ibuprofen for pain. She was referred to the Breast Health ███ for followup and presents for same. She reports that since being seen at █████████ her husband has been changing the dressings on her left breast. There has been a minimal amount of drainage noted. The dressing was most recently changed last p.m. She reports that her pain at the time of her I&D was 10 on a scale of 1-10. The pain has decreased since that time. She reports some decrease in the extent of the redness noted. She denies any nipple discharge, pulling, tugging, or dimpling.

## Breast Care - Outpt Record

\* Preliminary Report \*

### PAST BREAST HISTORY
She does report a history of a previous mastitis while nursing approximately 3 years ago, however, denies abscess formation.

### MAMMOGRAM HISTORY
She reports she did have a mammogram at ████████ in ████ in November, which was reportedly within normal limits and ultrasound as noted above.

### GYNECOLOGICAL HISTORY
The patient is P4, G4, however, 1 of her children died in the neonatal period. She is not currently using a form of contraception, however, reports LMP January 3, ████ with normal amount and duration of flow.

### FAMILY HISTORY
Negative for breast, ovarian, colon, or prostate cancer.

### CURRENT MEDICATIONS
1. Bactrim DS 2 tabs twice daily.
2. Ibuprofen 200 mg every 4-6 hours as needed for pain.
3. Oxycodone 5 mg, 1-2 tablets every 8 hours as needed for pain.
4. Tylenol 500 mg every 6 hours as needed for pain.

### PAST MEDICAL HISTORY
The patient does report an allergy to vancomycin. She denies other antibiotic allergies. She does report a history of anxiety and depression and a history of gallstones as well as hypertension. She additionally has had gestational diabetes. She denies other chronic or acute disease.

### PAST SURGICAL HISTORY
C-section times 2 in ████ and ████ as well as an umbilical hernia repair.

### REVIEW OF SYSTEMS
A 14-system review of systems was completed. Please refer to the Breast Health ████ Patient Intake Form.

GASTROINTESTINAL: The patient does report some cramping and constipation secondary to current pain medications. She denies other acute complaints at this time, other than those associated with the current breast problem.

### Breast Care - Outpt Record

* Preliminary Report *

### SOCIAL HISTORY
The patient does not work. She is married. Her husband accompanies her today. She denies exposure to chemicals or radiation. She is a nonsmoker. She drinks 1 to 2 caffeinated beverages per day, 2 servings of high-fat food. She does not drink alcohol. She exercises with caring for her children and cleaning house.

### PHYSICAL EXAMINATION
VITAL SIGNS: Weight is 166. Blood pressure 110/66, pulse 84 and regular, temp is 36.6.
GENERAL: Extremely pleasant, cooperative, however, somewhat anxious Hispanic female in no acute distress who is communicating through an interpreter this date. Her husband also accompanies her today and he does understand English.
HEENT: Normocephalic. Sclerae anicteric. Conjunctivae clear.
NECK: Supple, no nodes.
LUNGS: Completely clear throughout.
HEART: Regular rate and rhythm without audible murmur.
BREASTS: Asymmetric in appearance, the left larger than the right. There is a large, approximately 7-cm area of a circumareolar erythema and I&D site with packing. There is no erythema in the right breast. The packing from the left breast wound was removed revealing an approximate 2-cm wound with no visible exudate at this time. There is a minimal amount of exudate on the dressing. There is an area of thickness in the left breast measuring 7 x 5 cm, extending from the 7 o'clock position in the medial area of the breast to the 3 o'clock position in the lateral aspect of the breast. There is thickening in the subareolar area.

The left breast was prepped with Betadine and the wound repacked with half-inch gauze. Although this was a somewhat painful procedure, the patient tolerated the procedure well. The wound was then covered with 4x4s and secured in place.

### DIAGNOSTIC STUDIES
Ultrasound results as noted above. The previous mammogram is unavailable on today's exam.

### ASSESSMENT
████-year-old female with a long-standing history of an abscess in the left breast with I&D completed on January ██████

### PLAN
1.    I have discussed  with ████████████ who will plan on seeing her tomorrow at the

## Breast Care - Outpt Record

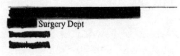

\* Preliminary Report \*

 Cancer Care Alliance at 4:30.

2.      will continue on her Bactrim.  I have added in Augmentin 875,1 twice daily for 10 days.  I have asked her to take at least 2 doses of her Augmentin today.  We have discussed the use of her pain medications and using the Oxycodone judiciously.

1.      We have discussed that GI upset is a common side effect with Augmentin, however, if she develops a rash, she should discontinue the medication and continue with her Bactrim as previously noted.

**Signature Line**

Surgery Dept

2406150

## Notes

1. T. Delbanco, et al., "OpenNotes: Doctors and Patients Signing On," *Annals of Internal Medicine* 153 (2010): 121–25.
2. Ibid.
3. Ibid.
4. T. Delbanco, et al., "Inviting Patients to Read their Doctors' Notes: A Quasi-experimental Study and a Look Ahead," *Ann Intern Med* 157 (2012): 464.
5. Ibid.
6. Ibid.
7. Ibid.
8. http://www.bidmc.org/News/Around-BIDMC/2013/August/OpenNotes .aspx.
9. T. W. Feeley and K. I. Shine (eds.), "Access to the Medical Record for Patients and Involved Providers: Transparency through Electronic Tools," *Annals of Internal Medicine* 155 (2011): 853–54.
10. http://www.healthcareitnews.com/news/cleveland-clinic-opens-emr-patients?topic=08,18.
11. https://www.myhealth.va.gov/mhv-portal-web/anonymous.portal?_nfpb =true&_nfto=false&_pageLabel=faqsHome#MHVFeatures.
12. http://www.cobar.org/index.cfm/ID/226/subID/1348/CITP/Medical-Records/.
13. http://www.fhima.org/NewsAndHotTopics_Homepage/Press%20Release %20-%20New%20Physician%20Medical%20Record%20Copy%20Fees %20Now%20In%20Effect.pdf.
14. http://www.health.ny.gov/publications/1443/.

# CHAPTER 4

# Using Video Games to Improve Health

*Sara Solovitch*

## Introduction

If philanthropy represents society's venture capital fund for ideas, the Foundation's pioneer portfolio is its high-risk investment pool. The chance of being awarded a grant or series of grants is relatively low and the chance of having a successful program is even lower, but when there is success, it can be a blockbuster.

One of the potential breakthrough ideas that the Foundation sought to nurture through its pioneer team was the use of video games to improve health. Although this may strike some readers as counterintuitive—don't video games lead kids to sit on the couch all day and grow fat?—in fact, games can be used to help people become healthier. As Sara Solovitch reports in this chapter, the Foundation's pioneer team worked to bring the gaming and research communities closer together and invested in research on the effectiveness of video games for health, primarily through a program called *Health Games Research*.

Sara Solovitch, an award-winning journalist and former reporter for *The Philadelphia Inquirer* and *The San José Mercury-News*, has been a frequent contributor to the *Robert Wood Johnson Foundation Anthology* series. She is completing a book on stage fright, to be published in 2015.

—w— A car races along a twisting, turning road, and your job is to stay the course with just the click of your left thumb. Your right thumb is responsible for shooting down one of those pesky road signs that pops up every few seconds. It's multitasking, it's unnerving, and it's more than just a little bit fun.

The game is the brainchild of Adam Gazzaley, a neuroscientist better known for his academic research on cognitive decline in older adults—namely, how memory impairment occurs as people become increasingly susceptible to distraction. Gazzaley, who holds both a medical degree and a doctorate in neuroscience, is director of the Neuroscience Imaging Center at the University of California, San Francisco, and he had long wondered whether this kind of cognitive impairment was reversible. Over the years, he developed tests to find out. But the tests were so boring that he doubted if anyone would ever take them with the kind of attention and focus required to actually change brain patterns.

Then one day it occurred to him: "Oh, that's what *games* do. That's why people play games and why kids don't even get up to go to the bathroom. Because they're so involved in them."

That epiphany gave birth to *NeuroRacer*, a video game—the one with those pesky road signs—that draws on a mix of cognitive skills, including attention focusing, task switching, and working memory (the ability to hold information in mind). Gazzaley was immediately convinced that he had come up with something valuable, but nobody was interested in bankrolling the idea—not until 2009, when the Robert Wood Johnson Foundation invested $287,000 in his project. That modest investment, part of a larger program called Health Games Research, dedicated to exploring the role of gaming in health, allowed Gazzaley to study the effects of *NeuroRacer* on forty-six participants between the ages of sixty and eighty-five. He and his colleagues monitored brain activity and observed eye positions over four weeks of game play, and concluded that the aging game players showed dramatic improvement in multitasking abilities. Their performances were not just better than those of twenty-year-olds who played the game only once; they demonstrated significant improvement in tasks completely separate from the game, tasks that tested them on their sustained attention and working memory, both critical assets for multitasking.

"And that's the holy grail of our field," says Gazzaley, whose results were published in the September 5, 2013, issue of the journal *Nature*. The article reflected the exuberance of its author. "These findings," it reported, "highlight the robust plasticity of the prefrontal cognitive control system in the ageing brain, and provide the first evidence, to our knowledge, of how a custom-designed video game can be used to assess cognitive abilities across the lifespan, evaluate underlying neural mechanisms, and serve as a powerful tool for cognitive enhancement." [1]

The game proved a big hit for Gazzaley, a striking man who, with his shock of white hair and cultivated stubble, looks more like a Hollywood producer than a university neurologist. He had been fiddling around with the idea for a couple of years, inspired in part by friends who were top designers and programmers at San Francisco-based LucasArts Entertainment Company. "We were like a mutual admiration society," says Gazzaley. "I'm like, 'Wow, you build video games.' And they're like, 'Wow, you study the brain and that's awesome.' We thought what each other did was impressive and fascinating, and we always thought it would be fun to work together some day."

That opportunity arose when, grant in hand, he took the prototype of his game to his friends. They then designed the artwork, programmed the software, and threw in a few bells and whistles, all largely for free. "They got a total of five thousand dollars," he says. "Little stipends. These guys are high-paid professional video-game developers; some of them didn't even take it. They said, 'I already have my job, this is my volunteer work.'"

While other health games have floundered because of poor design, *NeuroRacer* created a buzz. "I would say it's 'fun,'" Gazzaley says, his fingers making air quotes. "But barely. We didn't have the funding or the time to make it *really* fun. That wasn't even the goal. The goal was to make it fun enough for people to do."

The real fun came later. A good two years before the game made the cover story in *Nature*, it attracted several million dollars in venture capital money and spun off into a commercial company. Today, Boston-based Akili Interactive Labs is run and staffed by Gazzaley's friends, the onetime LucasArts developers. Gazzaley is Akili's chief science advisor. And the game that was originally designed for older people has been repurposed—complete with new story, music, and art—into a product for young people with attention deficit hyperactivity disorder (ADHD). That repurposing was at least partly financial: ADHD is "a massive global issue," Gazzaley says, with a potentially enormous payoff.

Akili has submitted the game, renamed *Project:EVO*, to the US Food and Drug Administration, seeking its approval as a therapy device that doctors can prescribe for young patients with ADHD. The company is also branching out to medical disorders beyond ADHD. If Akili has calculated correctly, video games may become a major therapeutic device for some of the most intractable health problems of the modern age.

## —∿— The Potential of Games to Improve Health

This is a story of a still emerging field, one with enormous potential to revolutionize health care. It is also a story of great optimism and almost equally great frustration. Though most observers believe that gaming has an inevitable future role in health care, its adoption has been slow and its promises as yet unfulfilled.

Video games today wield more economic clout than movies, and their power is expected to grow exponentially, from $63 billion in global revenues in 2012 to a projected $87 billion in 2017.[2] In the United States, the best-selling game of 2010, *Call of Duty: Black Ops*, generated more sales on its first day than any book, record album, or movie in history, including *Star Wars*. As the industry changes and matures, so does the profile of its players. According to the Entertainment Software Association, today's game players include more women over eighteen than boys under eighteen. More than 50 percent of households have a dedicated game console, and more than half of American parents view game playing as a positive influence on their children's lives.[3]

Back in 2004, when the Robert Wood Johnson Foundation made its first foray into the field, the potential implications for health care appeared enormous but still largely untapped. There were a handful of simulation games for training health professionals, some virtual reality programs for anxiety disorders, a few cognitive health games, some biofeedback programs, and some promising games in the pipeline. One of the latter, *Re-Mission*, released in 2006 by the nonprofit HopeLab in Redwood City, California, has been highly effective in helping young cancer patients manage their symptoms and comply with chemotherapy and other treatment regimens. This is no small feat for a video game—or even for a structured treatment plan, for that matter.

But finding the next big health game has proved difficult. Health games today reflect but a fraction of the industry share; their research and development budgets barely approach $100 million—a mere pittance, considering that developing graphics for a single game for Microsoft's Xbox can easily cost $10 million. Bringing the power of gaming to health is a stubbornly elusive endeavor. Consider the fate of Expresso Fitness, a Silicon Valley company that builds videos and simulation software to enhance a player's experience of riding on an Expresso stationary bike. The game was designed to entice people into exercising longer in order to lose weight and gain strength and endurance.

The company attracted $44 million from venture capital firms, but, according to the *Wall Street Journal*, the financiers exited in 2009 when the recession undermined the market plans and gyms decided they didn't need the equipment after all.

"Investing in individual games or sensors is kind of a crap shoot," says William Rosenzweig, managing partner at Physic Ventures, one of the investors in Expresso Fitness. "It's very fad-oriented. You don't know which one is going to take off . . . for games to be enduring in light of the rate of technological change, they have to be threaded into your life. I don't know how you figure out which game is going to be Monopoly."

## —〰— Games for Health: Bringing the Health and Video Game Communities Together

Health gaming got a shot in the arm when the pioneer portfolio of the Robert Wood Johnson Foundation made an exploratory investment in 2004. Then a newly created program team, pioneer, was charged with seeking out unconventional, breakthrough approaches to health care problems.

Paul Tarini, a senior program officer at the Foundation who was a leader of the pioneer team, recognized a medium with potential, one that could be customized for different audiences and platforms. "At that time, there wasn't much intersection between the games space and the health space," says Tarini. "What existed were games to train professionals to do their jobs, and a big chunk of that was in the military. But no one was thinking how to use games in a therapeutic setting. We saw that when kids played games, they would spend a lot of time with the game, and that they were able to retain a lot of information. It seemed to be very 'sticky.' So we wondered how to use games as a supportive therapy to facilitate behavior change."

Hoping to stimulate interest in video games for health, the pioneer portfolio made an initial grant of $250,000 in 2004 to Digitalmill, a games consulting firm in Portland, Maine. The grant was intended to explore the intersection between two disparate worlds—the world of video games and the world of health and health care—and to accelerate research. Ben Sawyer, who ran Digitalmill, had the ideal background for the job. A game developer and cofounder of the Serious Games Initiative at the Woodrow Wilson International Center for Scholars in Washington, D.C., he had spent the previous five years seeking to expand the use of games beyond entertainment.

Before 2004, says Sawyer, people were "mostly doing stuff on their own or getting small bits and pieces of grants." Now, with his pioneer seed money, Sawyer expanded the Games for Health Project, an organization charged with building the field through meetings and social networking, and convened the annual Games for Health Conference, where health policy researchers and health care providers could meet with game developers and entrepreneurs. The games community needed to understand that health was a viable segment of the market, one driven by evidence-based research. And the health community needed to appreciate the potential benefits of games to patients and consumers.

Between 2004 and 2013, the Games for Health Conference grew from 120 researchers, health professionals, and game developers to more than 400. The subject matter was just as diverse as the attendees. Presentations ranged from how to use games to deliver health messages to gaming strategy for post-traumatic stress disorder, stroke rehabilitation, and anxiety reduction.

As Sawyer had envisioned, the conferences generated new collaborations and projects. One of the most noteworthy began when Doris C. Rusch, currently the director of the MIT Game Lab, gave a presentation about a game she was working on to help the families of addicts understand addiction. A Harvard psychiatrist in the audience, T. Atilla Ceranoglu, approached her afterward and asked if her game could be modified for depression. So was born the game *Elude*. "It's a great example of what can happen if you just get people in a room together," says Sawyer. "Our goal all along has been to build some nexus to the space."

With that in mind, he published white papers and gave presentations that defined the concept of games for health, listed notable health-related games, and laid out ideas for the field's future. Sawyer also posed provocative questions: Was it reasonable to think that video games could change health care? Would providers use them? Would insurance companies get behind them? Could gaming prove an effective way to change behavior and not just attitude? Did the words *health* and *video games* even belong in the same sentence?

## —∿— Health Games Research: Building a Body of Knowledge

By 2007, satisfied that this was a field deserving attention, the Foundation authorized $8.25 million for the University of California, Santa Barbara (UCSB) to establish a national program called Health Games Research: Advancing Effectiveness of Interactive Games for Health. The program was designed to build a body of knowledge; to determine whether health games could in fact change health care; and to advance innovation, design, and effectiveness. Of the total grant, $4 million was set aside for disbursal to twenty-one research projects around the country. The research was to concentrate on games, such as Adam Gazzaley's *NeuroRacer*, that help prevent or manage chronic illnesses, rather than on games that, say, train clinicians. The remaining funds paid for staffing, technical assistance to the twenty-one projects, communications, a Web site, and a database of health-related video games. Digitalmill received about $750,000 to continue its annual conference and research.

The Health Games Research program was directed by Debra Lieberman, a widely recognized media researcher at UCSB's Institute for Social, Behavioral, and Economic Research and a lecturer in the University's Department of Communications. Lieberman has devoted much of her career to the study of digital media and games as a tool for learning and behavior change. Fresh out of college in 1973, she received a fellowship to Harvard University's Graduate School of Education, where she helped *Sesame Street* researchers and producers in the development of new TV programs for children. In the early 1990s, as vice president of research at a Silicon Valley health software company, she helped develop Super Nintendo video games to motivate health behavior change in patients with Type 1 diabetes and asthma.

Early results of Super Nintendo games showed promise. A randomized, controlled study reported that the diabetes game was especially effective for children between eight and sixteen. Before playing the game, the kids in the study averaged two-and-a-half diabetes-related urgent care and emergency visits per year. "Six months later they had dropped down to an average of one-half visits per child per year," Lieberman says. "That's a 77 percent drop and at least a two thousand dollar reduction in medical costs per child per year. We thought we had a business, anticipating that health plans would buy our games and give them to their members to improve health and reduce costs. . . . But we discovered that in the 1990s the medical world was not yet ready for this."

Health Games Research awarded its grants on the basis of a game's meeting at least one of two prerequisites: it had to require physical activity, or it had to enhance a player's health-related knowledge, skills, attitudes, and social support. Under the Foundation's guidelines, no grant could exceed $300,000, a decision that was controversial but closely reasoned; the projects were chosen to focus on studying health games, not developing them. Also, no more than 25 percent of a grantee's budget could be spent on game development. "The bottom line is that we needed more well-designed and robust research studies in our field, and it was important not to cut corners in research support," Lieberman says. "For the health care community, the biggest hurdle to embracing games has been a dearth of peer-reviewed data that provide a standard of proof that health games really do work."

In addition to Gazzaley's project, grantees included:

- Researchers at Georgetown University in Washington, D.C., who measured weight loss among obese and overweight African American adolescents after playing Nintendo's Wii Active exergame. The seven-month experiment examined physiological, social, and cognitive outcomes, and compared youths who played competitively with those who played cooperatively. The results, while mixed, suggested considerable value in sharing difficult goals with a teammate, as the youths who played cooperatively lost weight; those who played competitively did not.[4]

- Students and professors at Teachers College, Columbia University in New York, who developed and evaluated a smoking reduction game called *Lit2Quit*. A player breathes into the microphone of a cell phone, which then uses sound, color, images, rewards, and feedback responses to control breathing and mimic the stimulant and relaxant effects of smoking. The idea is to get smokers who are trying to quit to reach for this five-minute game instead of a cigarette. The results have not yet been published.

- Researchers at Indiana University, Bloomington, who studied an alternate reality game designed to promote physical activity and healthy lifestyles among college freshmen. *BloomingLife: The Skeleton Chase* involves an interactive story that unfolds over the course of eight weeks, using a variety of media (e-mail, Web sites, phone calls from fictional characters, physiological monitoring) and real-world physical and mental challenges. Preliminary results show that collaborative and social gaming positively influence physical activity.

- Researchers at the University of Vermont, Burlington, who studied whether a biofeedback video game could improve cystic fibrosis patients' use of inhaled medicines and breathing exercises and awareness of their respiratory status. The research team developed the breath biofeedback game

in collaboration with patients. Results indicated
that the game helps give adolescent patients
the autonomy they crave, using recreational
activities to support treatment demands.

## —⟋⟍— Face Station: A Game for Autistic Children

*FaceStation,* funded under the Health Games Research program, is
a suite of arcade-style games designed to improve face perception
skills in eight- to seventeen-year-olds with an autism spectrum disorder. Developed and tested at the Center for Autism Research
at The Children's Hospital of Philadelphia, this series of games
appeared a perfect fit for its target audience, since many young
people whose conditions fall on the autism spectrum share an
all-consuming interest in technology and computer games. The
goal of *FaceStation* was to help them read facial expressions and
distinguish one face from another; players would do so by linking
rewards to the close observation of faces, something autistic kids
would typically rather avoid.

In fact, however, the idea proved more difficult to carry out
than the researchers had anticipated. The preparation itself was
a massive job, entailing the collection and editing of some one
thousand photos of more than a hundred actors, every image
taken at a different angle and employing a different facial expres-
sion, be it angry, happy, sad, or surprised. Game development
and pilot testing proved so expensive that the grant's budget
was entirely depleted before tests for clinical efficacy could even
*begin.* The game designers and the scientists negotiated at length
over the acceptable levels of violence and "fun"—as opposed
to "training"—that could be included. Though they eventually
reached an agreement, the results were mixed. *FaceStation* fell
short of the level of sophistication that young people have come
to expect from video games, and while the treatment schedule
required near-daily game play, the youths' parents frequently had
to cajole them into playing.

Despite such challenges, the feedback proved tantalizing enough that Robert Schultz, director of the Center for Autism Research, decided to take the project to the next step. Drawing on his own internal funding, he launched a new study. A group of youths with autism would be given a nasal spray of oxytocin minutes before playing the game. The autism community has pinned much hope on oxytocin, a naturally occurring hormone that is released in the body during childbirth, lactation, and socialization. Research labs around the country are currently testing it on autistic children and teens, with early results showing increased social interaction and improved social communication skills. Scientists at the Center for Autism Research are similarly excited about the hormone's potential, but they believe it needs to be combined with a structured treatment plan—such as a video game.

Which is why, one morning in late summer 2013, a fourteen-year-old boy from New Jersey happened to be driving with his mother to Philadelphia. Jay is a handsome boy whose life revolves around video games. Once he arrived at the clinic, he stared out the window, unengaged, as he answered a graduate student's endless research questions. Then Jay asked a question of his own: "What's the nasal spray for?"

"Good question," replied the graduate student. "It's to see if it helps kids play games better." That was accurate enough. If oxytocin is as promising as hoped, game players will recognize faces much faster than they would just by playing the game without the oxytocin.

"I never thought I'd need medication to make me play better," said Jay, his eyes still trained toward the window. He has a dry wit and clearly enjoys making people laugh, despite the fact that he rarely makes eye contact.

After his mother sprayed puffs of the hormone in his nasal passages, Jay was soon clicking away—matching smiling faces, perturbed faces, and frowning faces in a series of games with names like *Dr. Face's Potion Shop* and *The Adventures of Pennsylvania Jones*. Jay clicked and clicked as computerized pings signified reward.

"He spends hours and hours on computer games," said his mother, watching. "It's really out of control. He doesn't want to go outdoors, he doesn't want to go anywhere or do anything. All he wants is to play video games. He's not an outdoor child."

"Maybe if you took the TV outside," Jay said drolly, his eyes never leaving the screen.

Gaming itself holds no special interest for the autism Robert Schultz. "I'm not fascinated with games, I'm fascinated with treatment," he says. That is why Schultz intends to stay involved with games. Recently contacted by Akili Interactive Labs, the company launched by Adam Gazzaley's game, Schultz found their offer an enticing one. "It's an extremely powerful-looking group," he says. "The people they have backing them are very esteemed. Plus, they want to develop something for autism, which is where I want to make my impact."

## —∼— A Burgeoning, Struggling Field

By setting its considerable footprint in the gaming world, the Robert Wood Johnson Foundation has given it a measure of validity. Suddenly, the phrase "health games" no longer sounds like an oxymoron. "You can call it anecdotal," says Digitalmill's Ben Sawyer, "but I've heard it a million times. People from health insurers, government agencies, large bureaucracies—when I've called, I get my calls returned. They tell me, 'Half the reason I can talk to you is that the Robert Wood Johnson Foundation is signaling this is worth taking a look at.'"

In 2006, the Centers for Disease Control and Prevention (CDC) sponsored a conference that included sessions on health games, after which it encouraged some of its employees to develop game ideas. One employee, Dan Baden, a physician and the associate director for external partner outreach and connectivity in the CDC's Office for State, Tribal, Local, and Territorial

Support, took the bait and began exploring the use of games to advance public health.

In 2011, he attended Ben Sawyer's Games for Health Conference. "If I hadn't gone to that conference, I wouldn't have received all the invitations to speak that I do today," says Baden, who now spends a dedicated portion of his time developing health games for the CDC. "I've been able to educate others on the amount of activity going on in this field. If I say that the Robert Wood Johnson Foundation is in this field, it carries weight."

Baden is part of a loose network of aspiring game developers within the CDC. Most of their products are training games, intended for internal use, but some are available externally. One, *Solve the Outbreak*, gives players the chance to explore disease outbreaks and learn what it is like to be an epidemiologist. Another teaches coal miners how to evacuate mines safely during emergencies.

Baden is particularly proud of a game he designed that helps primary care physicians understand the impact of public health on clinical practice. Developed to support the US Department of Health and Human Service's "Million Hearts" initiative, a national plan to prevent a million heart attacks and strokes by 2017, it is a basic time-management game. As the clock ticks, the number of patients in the waiting room builds, putting pressure on the player who has fifteen to twenty seconds to address each patient's heart disease risk factors. "The kicker," says Baden, "is that after you complete a level, you can spend points to implement health policies—like smoke-free air—and this will decrease the percentage of future patients who smoke. The point is to show clinicians that public health policy has the ability to improve the health of their patients and make them easier to treat, which in turn makes physicians' lives easier."

The National Institute on Drug Abuse also got involved, funding a few video games as tools for treating substance abuse. One, a virtual reality game, tosses virtual cigarette packs into virtual trashcans. Another, a prevention education game called *Media*

*Detective,* teaches elementary-aged children to spot hidden elements in ads that may encourage drug and alcohol use. A series of games, *Reconstructors,* teaches adolescents about the biological and social impact of drug abuse. Middle school students learn how classes of drugs affect the body, especially the nervous system, and are encouraged to develop negative attitudes toward drug use.

"Provided the games are appropriately targeted," says Jessica C. Chambers, program official/health science administrator at the National Institute on Drug Abuse, "video games have the potential to have a positive impact on behavior change among substance abusers, particularly youth substance abusers. Whereas many youths report a dislike of, and discomfort with, the one-on-one format of traditional behavioral substance abuse treatment, they seem to be very attracted to technology. And it is pervasive in their culture."

Despite these bursts of investment and experimentation, the burgeoning field continues to struggle. Consider Humana's investment in gaming. In 2008, the nation's fourth-largest health insurance company rolled out *Horsepower Challenge*, an exergame that it pilot-tested among a group of one hundred sixth-graders at five public schools in Louisville, Kentucky. The children were given wireless pedometers and encouraged to walk. All their steps were recorded and uploaded to power a networked video game. The more steps they took, the more power they had to play the game.

The game proved a huge success. After a four-week trial, Humana reported a 13 percent increase across all five schools in the number of steps, with 53 percent of the kids reporting that they had begun to exercise at home with their families. Humana announced plans to take the game to twenty additional cities, which it did in 2009 and 2010. And then, one day, the game was gone. So was the company's gaming division and Innovation Center. The experiment was over.

Today, Humana partners with the video game company Ubisoft. "It is fair to say that we have shifted some of the focus of our community health and well-being initiatives to 'live play,'" says Kate Marx, a company spokeswoman. "These include pedal buses that we deployed at our national conventions during 2012; our WalkIt Challenge with the PGA Tour; and the playgrounds we are building across the country with KaBOOM!"

From the beginning, Kaiser Permanente has taken a more cautious approach. "When we look at childhood obesity, our message to parents is that kids need less screen time, not more," says David Sobel, medical director of patient education and health promotion at The Permanente Medical Group. "Yet, newer approaches to applying gaming to changing behavior can be both more physically and mentally engaging—especially when compared to traditional forms of health education, such as reading materials and classes."

Sounding a little envious, Sobel says that what he finds exciting about the people who design games "is that they are as much behavior folks as they are tech people. When health information is well designed and engaging, the focus is on the content and engagement strategies first, and then the technology of how to deliver it. Sometimes the missing ingredient is how to mix them together to be engaging and fun. Games are designed to manipulate and influence people. The health game designers understand a lot about what drives human behavior."

It is not surprising, then, that Kaiser Permanente has begun testing the gaming waters. In 2008, it established the Innovation Fund for Technology, a program charged with exploring and developing new technologies. As of 2013, it had funded three health games, one of which, *Dr. Hero*, was the idea of Sonia Soo Hoo, a Kaiser Permanente obstetrician/gynecologist who was inspired in part by her game-playing daughters. Soo Hoo's game, intended for training OB/GYN care teams and residents, and developed with help from a professional gaming company, is now being widely used throughout the organization's Northern California region.

## —∿— Video Games for Health—An Oxymoron?

The mere mention of "health video games" tends to raise eyebrows. In the public's mind, sitting in front of a video screen is often associated with negative health outcomes, from obesity to antisocial behavior. In 2009, President Obama gave a speech before the American Medical Association in which he said parents should take responsibility for their children's health by "raising our children to step away from video games and spend more time playing outside." In 2011, the American Academy of Pediatrics issued a policy statement—its first in twelve years on the subject—discouraging television and other screen time for children under two. In doing so, it cited the lack of evidence supporting developmental benefits and pointed to potential adverse health and developmental effects on young children.

But now a growing discussion among researchers, educators, neuroscientists, doctors, and policy analysts is questioning that perspective. Neurologists are quick to note that while every activity, be it reading a book or playing the trombone, changes the brain, video games are somehow "different." Their effectiveness lies in the way they activate the brain's reward system, strengthening the synaptic connections of neural circuits in much the same way that pumping iron builds muscles. "Yes, some video games are sedentary," says Health Games Research program director Debra Lieberman. "But we do a lot of sedentary things, such as reading or going to the movies, and no one says that these pastimes are sedentary and therefore bad. Reading, movies, and game playing should be done in moderation and everyone should get plenty of physical activity, social interaction, work time, and so on. Don't blame video games . . . there are plenty of times during the day when you are not going to be jumping around anyway."

Moreover, says Lieberman, citing games for malaria prevention, alcohol relapse, and stroke rehabilitation, "games can improve prevention behaviors, healthy lifestyle behaviors, self care, adherence, disease self-management, clinical training, and delivery of care."

The arguments pro and con reflect not only the research but also personal experience. Jessie Gruman, the founder and president of the Center for Advancing Health in Washington, D.C., has argued that game designers are so far removed from the reality of sickness that they don't understand something basic: it can't be made "fun." A three-time cancer survivor since her diagnosis of Hodgkin's lymphoma at age twenty, Gruman, now sixty, took on the health gaming industry in February 2013 in an open letter directed at mobile health app developers.[5] Published on her organization's Web site, the letter detailed how, when she traded in her old phone for a new one, she realized she wasn't interested in loading "even a single one of the twenty-three health-related apps that I had carefully chosen and used from the old phone to the new." She wrote that her experience with these apps had left her feeling "ornery and impatient." Her letter went viral.

"Being a sick person is tedious, difficult, and boring," says Gruman, "and most people would rather spend less time thinking about it instead of playing a game about it. Like right now, I try to keep a food diary. But it takes me more time to write down what I eat than it does to eat it. I don't want to play a game. I already spend far too much time accommodating to my illness, resting from it, talking to people about it, transferring my records. Anything that adds to the burden of me doing it is just not going to work. Maybe a kid would one time play a game, but I just can't see it."

But to hear Carolyn Thomas tell it, video games aren't just for kids. Thomas, sixty-three, is a heart attack survivor who has become a big fan of the Nintendo Wii, using it to work out her frustrations, engage with family members, and get a punishing workout that leaves her gasping for breath and drenched with sweat. Like Gruman, Thomas has become a forceful patient advocate—in her case, both in her hometown of Victoria, British Columbia, and online, where her blog (www.myheartsisters.org)

has drawn more than a million followers worldwide since launching in 2009. She began developing her base after suffering a major heart attack, originally misdiagnosed as acid reflux, at age fifty-eight. A longtime distance runner, Thomas had never imagined herself as a cardiac patient: "I bought the stereotype that heart attacks happen to men. I thought a heart attack is when you clutch your chest and fall down unconscious. That's a sudden cardiac arrest; that's not a heart attack. Women can walk and talk and pick up the kids and cook dinner while they're having a heart attack."

After her recovery, Thomas found herself indignant over the lack of knowledge about women's cardiac health and the fact that women younger than fifty-five are seven times more likely to be misdiagnosed than men in a cardiac emergency. Determined to change that statistic, in 2008 she attended the WomenHeart Science & Leadership Symposium, a one-week education "boot camp" at the Mayo Clinic in Rochester, Minnesota.

Upon her return home, she lectured to small groups and launched a series of "Pinot & Prevention" parties intended to educate women on their risk of heart attacks. On her blog, she has touted the pleasures of boxing and ski jumping on the Wii with her grown daughter: "You stand on a little pad that senses your weight and balance. Then you have to crouch down and leap up. It doesn't sound like much, but holy moly, the next day my daughter and I were paralyzed.... I go to regular physical fitness classes at the gym, but I never feel like I am dripping with sweat like I am at the end of an evening with my family. That's the beauty of the Wii. You're having fun. It tricks you into exercising."

## —∾— The Future: Promise and Frustration

Health games have come a long way. The field now has a bona fide community for networking and collaboration. "When we look at where the field was in, say, 2007, and where it is today," says the

Robert Wood Johnson Foundation's Paul Tarini, "our sense is that the notion that games can be used in health and health care is no longer novel but accepted."

Even so, health games have yet to be embraced by the major players in the commercial video game field. The problem appears to be the lack of a viable business model: Who will buy the games? Will insurance companies reimburse for their use? So far, these questions have no answers, but certainly no one expects that the business model for health games will mirror that of consumer games. It's highly unlikely that parents will line up to buy the latest version of *FaceStation* or even *NeuroRacer*, if it were available commercially, for a Christmas stocking. Video games are by their very nature consumable and disposable. Kids develop mastery, beat the game, and go on to the next one. This quality determines the business model.

The expectation for health games is, however, much higher than for commercial games. "A lot of health games are for kids with autism, kids with cancer," says managing director and global healthcare innovation leader Christopher Wasden of PricewaterhouseCoopers. "They're for very scary emotional challenges, and they try to teach kids through a game what to expect and how to improve their health. That more noble objective makes it more difficult than for other games to be successful. But how do you make it both noble and sustainable as a business? Given this dual requirement, to what extent should we have expectations that the health games segment can become very large?"

Wasden was recently engaged in an experiment designed to answer just these kinds of questions. An instructor at the University of Utah, he advised students in the Games4Health Challenge, a collaboration of the University's gaming/engineering program, business school, and health sciences center, to develop prototypes of health-related video games and smartphone applications. The ubiquity of smartphones and other mobile devices has altered the conversation on games, says Wasden. Up to now, most of the research on the efficacy of health games and apps has been conducted before the launch of smartphones.

"The reality," he says, "is that until smartphones came out, there weren't health games and apps that were engaging and effective. Most of the data were done on laptop and desktop computers, which make for clunky, cumbersome interfaces. The thing that makes games more engaging is putting them on a mobile platform."

For his part, Ben Sawyer, the founder of Games for Health, admits to being more than a little disappointed in the lack of progress. "We've watched entrepreneurs come and go and come again," he says. "We've watched foundations invest, retreat, and invest again. It's easy to create different pieces of games that have great opportunity, but the transfer of that to the health field is very difficult."

It's not that Sawyer has soured on the future of health games. It's just that he now sees that the transition will be much slower than he once expected. Yes, he says, a few games by independent developers are starting to make a dent—he cites one game designed to help people learn how to grieve, and another that tackles the subject of hormone replacement therapy. "But if you had asked me nine years ago if I would have seen more uptake by now, I would have said yes."

In addition to the nonexistent business model, Sawyer points to another challenge: Health games remain largely within the province of academia. They haven't begun to attract the interest of large game developers like Nintendo, Sony, and Electronic Arts. And without the big developers' skills in designing games that are fun, eye-popping, and engaging, their potential is limited.

"The important thing is, you can't let policy wonks, academics, and doctors design the game," says James Gee, a professor of literacy studies at Arizona State University and one of the most respected researchers in the field. While the content of a game may reside in academia, says Gee, the fun of the game—what makes it a game and not a straight-out lesson—lies with the game maker. "We're at the beginning of game developers making these games, and the academics have to step aside."

A longtime proponent of bringing the learning model of video games into the classroom, Gee sits on the advisory board of iCivics, a Web-based education project founded by retired US Supreme Court Justice Sandra Day O'Connor. He also sat on the national advisory committee to the pioneer portfolio as it wrestled with the programs it would fund. "I have the highest admiration for good games," says Gee. "Making a good game is an art form. There's no algorithm for it. People thought in the beginning that it would be really easy. But a good game has to have an interesting problem. And then it has to give a person an interesting way to solve it. Health is full of problems that don't have easy solutions."

By the end of the Health Games Research program in September 2013, it was clear that the Robert Wood Johnson Foundation's investment had helped bring credibility to a field where there had once been little. "Health games could have easily been a passing fancy that captured our imagination for a short while and then disappeared from memory or practice," says Bill Ferguson, the commissioning editor at Mary Ann Liebert, Inc., the academic publishing house that identified the niche for a dedicated journal, the *Games for Health Journal.* "The Robert Wood Johnson Foundation fostered the idea until it became mature enough to stand on its own feet."

But standing on its feet remains a problem. Now in its third year of publication, the *Games for Health Journal* has not been easy to sustain, according to Tom Baranowski, its current editor in chief. There has been a dearth of submissions, and reviewers still reject grants for video game research with belittling comments to the effect that "Games are the source of the problem of obesity. They should be completely restricted."

The Foundation's Paul Tarini remains hopeful, however. "If the question is whether there's a game that helps someone manage their diabetes, and that game is being used by five thousand diabetics—no, we haven't seen that level of use," he says. "But I think we're seeing more use and more acceptance of gaming in health and health care." Tarini points with pride to the pioneer team's early support of Digitalmill's Ben Sawyer, who helped launch the conversation. And he sees promise in the results of the Foundation's work with Adam Gazzaley and *NeuroRacer*. Commenting on the results of the *NeuroRacer* research published in *Nature*, he adds, "I think our timing was very good.

"It's always nice to see research get published in a high-quality journal. We take that as indication not only of the quality of the research, but that the research is relevant. If that research had been done ten years earlier, it may not have made it into *Nature*."

## Notes

1. A. Abbott, "Gaming Improves Multi-Tasking Skills," *Nature*, September 4, 2013. http://www.nature.com/news/gaming-improves-multitasking-skills-1.13674.
2. PWC, *Global Entertainment and Media Outlook: 2013–2017*, http://www. pwc.com/gx/en/global-entertainment-media-outlook/segment-insights/ video-games.jhtml.
3. Entertainment Software Association, *Essential Facts About the Computer and Video Game Industry*, 2012, http://www.theesa.com/facts/pdfs/ esa_ef_2013.pdf.
4. A. E. Staiano, "Adolescent Exergame Play for Weight Loss and Psychosocial Improvement," *Obesity*, 21(3), April, 2013.
5. http://www.cfah.org/blog/2013/an-open-letter-to-mobile-health-app-developers-and-their-funders#.UpQW92SidRY.

# Section Two
# Reducing Childhood Obesity

# CHAPTER 5

# The Robert Wood Johnson Foundation's Efforts to Reduce Childhood Obesity

*Stephen L. Isaacs, David C. Colby, and Amy Woodrum*

In the late 1990s and early 2000s, health researchers began to notice a growing phenomenon: Americans were putting on weight—and lots of it. The Centers for Disease Control and Prevention (CDC) had been depicting the phenomenon graphically in a series of maps in which states were colored according to their percentage of obese residents. Obesity was portrayed in fire-engine red. In 1994, there had not been a single state colored red. By 2000, eleven states were colored red, and by 2005, the numbers had become alarming: thirty-nine states were now colored red.

Serious health consequences accompany obesity, including increased risk of type 2 diabetes, heart attack and stroke, high blood pressure, and certain cancers, among others. By 2006, obesity was vying with tobacco as the nation's leading cause of death.[1] Moreover, obesity and its attendant health consequences

**Figure 5.1** Age-Adjusted Prevalence of Obesity, 1994

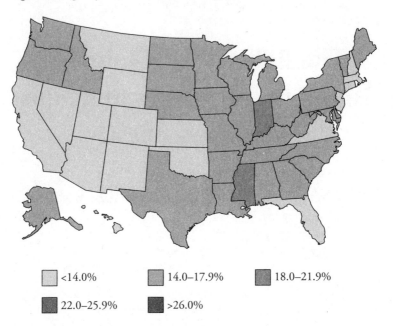

<table>
<tr><td>☐ <14.0%</td><td>▨ 14.0–17.9%</td><td>▨ 18.0–21.9%</td></tr>
<tr><td>▨ 22.0–25.9%</td><td>▨ >26.0%</td><td></td></tr>
</table>

*Source*: CDC's Division of Diabetes Translation. National Diabetes Surveillance System available at http://www.cdc.gov/diabetes/statistics

**Figure 5.2** Age-Adjusted Prevalence of Obesity, 2000

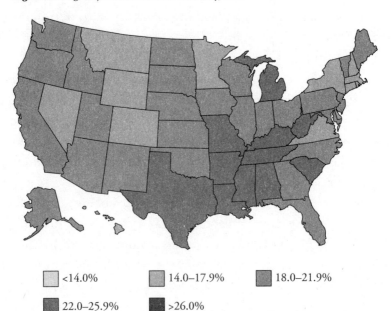

<table>
<tr><td>☐ <14.0%</td><td>▨ 14.0–17.9%</td><td>▨ 18.0–21.9%</td></tr>
<tr><td>▨ 22.0–25.9%</td><td>▨ >26.0%</td><td></td></tr>
</table>

*Source*: CDC's Division of Diabetes Translation. National Diabetes Surveillance System available at http://www.cdc.gov/diabetes/statistics

**Figure 5.3**  Age-Adjusted Prevalence of Obesity, 2005

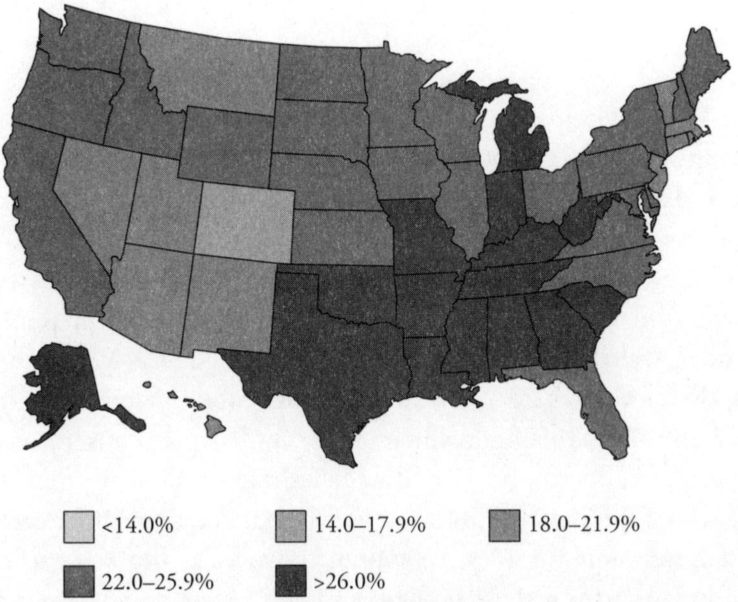

| | | |
|---|---|---|
| ☐ <14.0% | ☐ 14.0–17.9% | ☐ 18.0–21.9% |
| ☐ 22.0–25.9% | ☐ >26.0% | |

*Source*: CDC's Division of Diabetes Translation. National Diabetes Surveillance System available at http://www.cdc.gov/diabetes/statistics

were costing the nation an estimated $186 billion a year, or nearly 21 percent of annual medical spending in the United States.[2] And obesity was threatening the readiness of the Armed Forces. A study by an organization of retired military leaders found that at least 27 percent of young adults seventeen to twenty-four years of age were too fat to serve in the military, prompting retired US Army General Johnnie E. Wilson to state, "Child obesity has become so serious in this country that military leaders are viewing this epidemic as a potential threat to our national security."[3]

Moreover, obesity is not an equal-opportunity scourge. It disproportionately affects racial and ethnic minorities and poor, less educated people. Like smoking, obesity and its attendant diseases have come to characterize minorities and people in low socioeconomic classes.

By the end of the twentieth century, governments and foundations had begun shifting their priorities to address rising obesity. In 1997, the Paso del Norte Health Foundation in El Paso, Texas, began supporting the Coordinated Approach to Child Health (CATCH) program to reduce childhood obesity in elementary schools; as of 2010, the program had been expanded to more than seven thousand sites around the country. In 1999, The California Endowment funded Harold Goldstein, who had recently earned a Doctor of Public Health degree, to do a survey of the kinds of foods sold in public school vending machines; the survey revealed that 98 percent of the choices were unhealthy—chips, cookies, sodas, candy, and the like. The Endowment next funded programs to alert state legislators to obesity and diabetes rates in their districts; to increase access to healthy food and physical activity in selected California communities; to support advocates who were using information from these programs to effect state policies; and to make the media aware of obesity levels and their consequences in the state.

The federal government was paying attention as well. In 1996, the National Institutes of Health launched the Diabetes Prevention Program, which helped people lose weight as a way of preventing diabetes. Initial results of the program were published in the *New England Journal of Medicine* in 2002.[4] In 2001, the Surgeon General issued a landmark report entitled *The Surgeon General's Call to Action to Prevent and Decrease Overweight and Obesity*. Among those whom the report influenced was Risa Lavizzo-Mourey, at the time a senior vice president at the Robert Wood Johnson Foundation.

"Around the time I first joined the Foundation," says Lavizzo-Mourey, "the Surgeon General's report said that childhood obesity was a largely underappreciated problem, one that had been accelerating for nearly a decade and a half and that no one was taking on directly. Later, as I was preparing my first president's message, I remembered reading that report and thinking, 'Tackling obesity would be a perfect issue for the Robert Wood Johnson Foundation.'"

Although the Foundation had made some small obesity-related grants in the late 1990s,[5] and in the early 2000s had funded Active Living programs aimed at making the "built environment" more friendly to physical activity (see Will Bunch's report on the programs to improve the built environment in Chapter 7), the Foundation's work on childhood obesity prevention began in 2003 when Lavizzo-Mourey became the Foundation's president and CEO. She presented the Board with an Impact Framework to guide the Foundation's programming over the coming years, and one of its elements was addressing the growing epidemic of childhood obesity. Between 2003 and 2005, the Foundation planned its strategies to combat childhood obesity; launched one major new initiative, Healthy Eating Research; and piggybacked childhood obesity onto existing programs, such as Active for Life and the Diabetes Initiative.

In 2007, the Robert Wood Johnson Foundation made its well-publicized $500 million commitment to reversing the upward trend in childhood obesity. Drawing on the lessons from its past efforts, especially those to reduce smoking, the Foundation developed a wide-ranging strategy for addressing childhood obesity—one consisting of the following intersecting parts:

> *Develop a field of childhood obesity policy research*
> The Foundation developed its childhood obesity
> research programs based on the models of the
> Tobacco Policy Research and Evaluation Program
> and the Substance Abuse Policy Research Program.
> Enlisting some of the nation's leading researchers
> and seeding the work of new academic researchers
> who otherwise might have gone into different fields,
> the Foundation funded a new program, Healthy
> Eating Research, focused on food and nutrition,
> and changed the mandate of two existing research
> programs to focus on childhood obesity: Active

Living Research, which had been striving to make the built environment more friendly to physical activity, and Bridging the Gap, which had been monitoring substance abuse among students.

To make sure that the new field attracted black and Latino researchers, the Foundation also established the African American Collaborative Obesity Research Network and Salud America! The Robert Wood Johnson Foundation Research Network to Prevent Obesity Among Latino Children. In Chapter 6, Joe Alper discusses how the childhood obesity research field developed.

Additionally, the Foundation supported and collaborated with the Arkansas state government on research, tracking the progress of the state's obesity-reduction efforts by measuring the BMI (body mass index) of Arkansas schoolchildren. The Foundation also supported a series of highly influential research reports on childhood obesity by the Institute of Medicine, and joined with the CDC, National Institutes of Health, and US Department of Agriculture to form the National Collaborative on Childhood Obesity Research.

*Support community-level programs to promote physical activity and better access to healthy food*
Modeled in part after an earlier program, Active Living By Design (and managed by the same director), Healthy Kids, Healthy Communities has worked in fifty communities to bring about changes in the physical environment conducive to lowering children's weights—changes such as building bike paths, encouraging kids to walk to school, and making sure new street construction includes sidewalks. Marissa Miley examines the Healthy Kids, Healthy Communities Program in Chapter 9.

Under another community-focused program, Communities Creating Healthy Environments, advocacy organizations in twenty-three communities of color are incorporating the obesity issue into their broader social justice work—for example, by highlighting the lack of parks or access to fresh foods in poor neighborhoods as evidence of inequitable resource distribution, as well as barriers to healthy living.

The Foundation has also supported The Food Trust, a Philadelphia-based nonprofit, to attract supermarkets to inner cities and to encourage bodegas and corner grocery stores to sell fruits and vegetables. The work of The Food Trust was discussed by Will Bunch in Volume XV of the *Anthology*.

To reach young people where they are most likely to be found during the day, the Foundation joined forces with the Clinton Foundation and the American Heart Association to develop the Healthy Schools Program. Designed to engage administrators, teachers, vendors, and parents in increasing access to physical activity and healthier food for students and staff, this program is explored by Paul Jablow in Chapter 8.

*Bring the issue of childhood obesity and possible solutions to the attention of policymakers and the public*
As part of a major communications effort to bring the results of its research and community programs to the attention of policymakers and the public, the key people in the Foundation's work on childhood obesity—Risa Lavizzo-Mourey; James Marks, a senior vice president; and Dwayne Proctor, the leader of the childhood obesity team—spoke and wrote frequently about the importance of reducing childhood obesity and some of the ways that were proving effective in doing so. In addition, the Foundation generated wide publicity for the work of its grantees and gave its financial support to conferences, publications, and even television specials.

In another aspect of the communications effort, the Foundation funded the Trust for America's

Health to produce a series of annual report cards, *F as in Fat*, which called attention to the childhood obesity problem and scrutinized the efforts of governments and businesses to address it. And the Foundation's support of the Rudd Center for Food Policy & Obesity at Yale University triggered a number of highly publicized reports on the harmful effect of sodas and unhealthy food and the extent of advertising of sugar-filled products by the food and beverage industries.

The Foundation also collaborated with other important players to bring the problem of childhood obesity to the attention of policymakers and the public. In that regard, nothing generated more publicity than the *Let's Move!* campaign sponsored by First Lady Michelle Obama. The Foundation also participated in a consortium of childhood obesity prevention funders, initially called the Healthy Eating Active Living Convergence and later called simply the Convergence Partnership.

The Foundation has reached out to the business community by helping to organize two consortiums. The first is ChildObesity180, a consortium of obesity researchers and executives from the food, insurance, and pharmaceutical industries. The second is the Healthy Weight Commitment Foundation, which brings together leaders of sixteen leading packaged-food and beverage companies who pledged to remove 1.5 trillion calories from their products by 2015.

—⚉—

As it has done in the past with issues ranging from nurse practitioners and generalist medicine to end-of-life care and tobacco control, the Foundation seized an issue of importance and, using its reputation and its funds, helped shape the nation's response to the issue. In this case, the growing obesity epidemic was already in the health community's sights and, to a lesser extent, the public's as well. The Foundation was able to frame the problem in an understandable way (excess weight being the consequence of more calories coming in than going out); develop a body of research and a corps of researchers on the topic; collaborate with other foundations, government, and the private sector; launch an ambitious communications effort; develop a multifaceted strategy to raise consciousness about this growing epidemic with policy-makers and the public; and fund community- and school-based programs with the aim of changing the physical and social environments that were leading young people to gain weight.

Although the Foundation cannot take credit for them (it certainly made an important contribution, however), the encouraging news is that changes were visible by 2014. The nation was aware of the seriousness of childhood obesity and its health consequences, and governmental and private entities were taking steps to address it. Congress and the US Agriculture Department hotly debated the nutritional value of subsidized school meals in 2013. That same year, the American Medical Association named obesity as a disease. By 2014, the sale of sodas in public school vending machines, à la carte lines, and canteens had been banned in elementary schools by twenty-three states, in middle schools by twenty states, and in high schools by sixteen states. Moreover, McDonald's was advertising salads and at least one major food processor was trying to make healthier products.

Furthermore, by 2014 some areas of the country began to see signs of hope in obesity levels. The declines were few and geographically scattered, but, nonetheless, represented the first concrete signs of change. Many interpreted as a sign of progress a 2014 report published in the *Journal of the American Medical*

*Association* indicating that the prevalence of obesity among children aged two to five years decreased from 14 percent in 2003–2004 to just over 8 percent in 2011–2012.[6] The percent decline, however, is the subject of dispute.[7] Despite the need for confirmation by further studies, after decades of unhappy news, these signs of progress are welcome.

The discouraging news is that obesity remains a disease contracted primarily by poorer, less well-educated people and by racial and ethnic minorities. They have barely shared in the weight reductions seen by their more affluent, white neighbors.[8] The challenge for the future—a challenge that the Foundation is currently addressing—is making the gains in combating childhood obesity more equitable, so that all people, whatever their race, ethnicity, or class, can reap the benefits and enjoy healthier lives.

## Notes

1. G. Danaei, et al., "The Preventable Causes of Death in the United States: Comparative Risk Assessment of Dietary, Lifestyle, and Metabolic Risk Factors", *PLoS Medicine* 6, no. 4 (2009): e1000058.

2. J. Cawley, et al. "The Medical Care Costs of Obesity: An Instrumental Variables Approach," *Journal of Health Economics* 31 (2012): 219–30.

3. Mission: Readiness. *Too Fat to Fight*, 2010 http://www.missionreadiness .org/wp-content/uploads/MR_Too_Fat_to_Fight-11.pdf.

4. Diabetes Prevention Program Research Group, "Reduction in the Incidence of Type 2 Diabetes with Lifestyle Intervention or Metformin," *New England Journal of Medicine* 346 (2002): 393–403. The CDC took over the program in 2012.

5. These include grants for a supplement in *Pediatrics* on childhood obesity in 1997 and one on physical activity to prevent obesity in 1999. It also made a grant in 1999 to build a clearinghouse and resource center on increasing physical activity.

6. C. L. Ogden, et al., "Prevalence of Childhood and Adult Obesity in the United States, 2011–2012," *Journal of the American Medical Association* 311, no. 8 (2014): 806–14.

7. E. Oster, "Reports of Drop in Childhood Obesity are Overblown," http://fivethirtyeight.com/features/reports-of-a-drop-in-childhood-obesity-are-overblown/; A. C. Skinner and J. A. Skelton, "Prevalance and Trends

in Obesity and Severe Obesity among Children in the United States, 1999–2012," *JAMA Pediatrics* 168, no. 6 (2014m): 561–66, http://archpedi.jamanetwork.com/article.aspx?articleid=1856480.

8. An exception is Philadelphia, which has shown reductions in childhood obesity among black and Hispanic as well as white children.

# CHAPTER 6

# Building a Field of Childhood Obesity Research

*Joe Alper*

## Introduction

Among the earliest decisions the staff and Board of the new Robert Wood Johnson Foundation made in the early 1970s was that the Foundation would use *evidence* in determining how to address health problems. Evidence was to come from different sources: some from demonstration projects, some from evaluations, and some from research studies. This commitment to evidence and research has endured throughout the life of the Foundation. To a great extent, the Foundation's reputation rests on its commitment to rigorous research and evidence-based programming.

In the 1970s, the Foundation focused on gathering evidence about access to medical care: Who had problems gaining access? How much primary care did specialists provide? Did the use of the 911 phone number expand access to emergency care? By the 1980s, the Foundation had expanded its search for evidence to other topics, such as improvement of end-of-life care, support for homebound elderly people, and reduction in the cost of health care. In the 1990s, it funded research on policy and environmental levers to reduce smoking and other substance abuse. Research studies found, for example, that higher cigarette prices led to less smoking by teenagers and young adults. Furthermore, the Foundation put the results of research into practice. The coalitions built by the Campaign for Tobacco-Free Kids and the SmokeLess States National Tobacco Policy Initiative used the tobacco tax research to advocate for policy changes.

As Joe Alper notes, the Foundation's childhood obesity research has built on its tobacco-policy research experience. It created a new academic field of childhood obesity research, supported leading childhood obesity researchers, and attracted new researchers to the field; it also investigated policy levers that could increase access to healthy food and physical activity. Alper, an award-winning writer specializing in science and technology, has served as a contributing correspondent for *Science* and as a contributing editor of *Nature Biotechnology* and *Self* magazines. He has written or coauthored many chapters for the *Anthology* series.

Spend even a couple of minutes talking with James Sallis of the University of California at San Diego and you start having an almost irresistible urge to rush home and get all the children in your neighborhood together for a game of kick the can.

Talk for any length of time to Mary Story, formerly of the University of Minnesota and now with Duke University, or to Amelie Ramirez of the University of Texas Health Science Center at San Antonio, and you're ready to swear that you will never let your child touch another can of Coke or stick a straw in another pouch of Capri Sun ever again.

And after even a brief conversation with Frank Chaloupka of the University of Illinois at Chicago, or Marlene Schwartz at Yale University, or Shiriki Kumanyika of the University of Pennsylvania School of Medicine, it feels as though the very next thing you should do is call every member of your school board and demand to know why your local schools aren't serving healthier lunch foods or making physical education classes mandatory, and are instead allowing energy drink companies to advertise at high school sporting events.

Sallis, Story, Ramirez, Chaloupka, Schwartz, and Kumanyika come from a range of academic backgrounds, and each brings a unique perspective to the challenge of significantly reducing childhood obesity in America. They are the directors of six research programs the Robert Wood Johnson Foundation has funded to better understand the environmental, social, and policy issues that stand in the way of the nation making progress toward this goal; to identify the most effective approaches to overcoming obstacles; and to build a field of childhood obesity research. As such, they have played an important role in the Foundation's efforts to reverse the childhood obesity epidemic in the United States by 2015.

From a ten-thousand-foot view, the cause of the childhood obesity epidemic is straightforward—over the past forty years, kids have been consuming somewhere between 110 and

165 calories per day more than they've been burning. To put that in context, a twelve-ounce can of sugar-sweetened soda contains between 140 and 190 calories. On the activity side of the equation, substituting an hour of active play for an hour of television or video game playing reduces calorie expenditure by 92–102 calories per day. "When you look at the problem of childhood obesity from this simple perspective, it doesn't look to be that hard a problem to solve," says Tracy Orleans, senior scientist and distinguished fellow at the Foundation.

Orleans, along with Jim Marks, senior vice president, and Dwayne Proctor, leader of the Foundation's childhood obesity team, was a primary architect of the Foundation's strategy to develop a body of childhood obesity research and a corps of childhood obesity researchers. "But from any real-world perspective, you quickly find that there are many factors that influence what children eat and how active they are. As a result, it's going to take a broad strategy focused on those factors, rather than on individuals, to make an impact."

In 2000, well before the Foundation had recognized the importance of rising rates of obesity, it had initiated a series of programs designed to restructure the built environment in ways that would make it easier for people to walk, ride bikes, and in general become more physically active. The Active Living portfolio consisted of six programs, one of which was the Active Living Research program headed by Sallis, who was then at San Diego State University and is currently Distinguished Professor of Family and Preventive Medicine at the University of California, San Diego.

Active Living Research had three goals: to build the evidence base about environmental and policy correlates and determinants of physical activity; to build the capacity of researchers in a wide variety of fields to collaborate and conduct high-level studies to understand the links among environments, policies, and active living; and to communicate the findings of funded research to policymakers and practitioners whose work can change environments and policies. "The idea," explains Sallis, "was that Active Living Research would fund a range of large and small projects that together would support a new field of research on the environmental and policy influences on active living, with the goal of informing policy in a way that would have a positive impact on health. While the concept underlying this program—that the built environment can affect activity levels—was accepted in urban planning circles, what was really novel about the Foundation's entry into the field was that it was based on the idea that there was a connection between the built environment and adverse health consequences—in this case obesity."

In 2003, the Robert Wood Johnson Foundation was reorganized under the direction of newly appointed president and chief executive officer Risa Lavizzo-Mourey, and one of its top priorities became the prevention of childhood obesity. As part of that reorganization, the existing childhood obesity working group was reconfigured as a program team, incorporating and expanding the health and behavior team, which oversaw the Active Living portfolio. In 2007, the Foundation announced a $500 million, five-year commitment to reversing childhood obesity by 2015.

## —⟋⟍— Forging a Multipronged Research Agenda

The design of Active Living Research, as well as the others that made up the Active Living portfolio, was influenced heavily by the lessons the Foundation had learned from its Tobacco Policy Research and Evaluation Program. In particular, the Foundation's experience in the tobacco control arena demonstrated the importance of marrying research that identified what worked—for example, raising taxes on cigarettes to reduce tobacco use—with a concerted effort to spread the results of that research to policymakers at the national, state, and community levels.

That experience also buoyed the Foundation's growing interest in identifying policy and environmental strategies that would promote, at the population level, behavior changes relating to the challenge of reversing childhood obesity trends. "We came to the conclusion early on," says Marks, "that as with tobacco policies, there was not going to be a silver bullet that would prevent children from becoming overweight or obese, and that we would need to generate evidence supporting many different approaches to this problem."

The Foundation's childhood obesity team also realized that there was little in the way of research capacity existing to achieve these policy objectives. "We needed national programs that would not only conduct research that achieves these objectives," says Orleans, "but also do what we did in both our tobacco control and active living efforts—essentially create new research communities."

To that end, the Foundation repurposed two existing programs and rolled out four new ones that, together, would provide an evidence base on which to construct policies and programs to reduce childhood obesity:

- Active Living Research, an extension of the original program but with a new focus on childhood obesity, supported and shared research on the environmental and policy strategies that can promote daily physical activity for children and families. This program, which ended in December 2013, placed special emphasis on research related to children of color and lower-income children, as well as on policy influences that affect the ability of children and adolescents to be active.

- Healthy Eating Research conducts research on environmental and policy strategies with the potential to promote healthy eating among children; the program focuses especially on low-income and racial and ethnic populations at highest risk for obesity.

- Bridging the Gap is a program the Foundation funded originally in 1997 to assess the impact of policies, programs, and other environmental influences on adolescent alcohol, tobacco, and illicit drug use. It was redirected to identify the policy and environmental factors that have the greatest impact on diet, physical activity, and obesity among young people and to track trends and changes in these factors over time. Unlike Active Living Research and Healthy Eating Research, Bridging the Gap does not fund researchers external to the program.

- The Rudd Center for Food Policy & Obesity Research at Yale University assessed, critiqued, and publicized public policy and food industry practices related to nutrition and obesity. Foundation support of the program ended in November 2014.

- Salud America! The Robert Wood Johnson Foundation Research Network to Prevent Obesity Among Latino Children is a national online network of researchers, community group leaders, decision makers, and members of the public working together to support policy and environmental changes that can help reverse the Latino childhood obesity epidemic.

- The African American Collaborative Obesity Research Network (AACORN) is a collaboration of researchers, scholars-in-training, and community-based research partners dedicated to improving the quality and quantity of research to address weight-related health issues in African American communities.

Each program could be the subject of its own chapter in this volume. However, rather than recounting in detail all that has been learned from each program's effort, the following pages will illustrate the variety of ways in which these programs are generating evidence and using it to address the nation's childhood obesity epidemic.

**Figure 6.1** RWJF's Childhood Obesity Research Funding

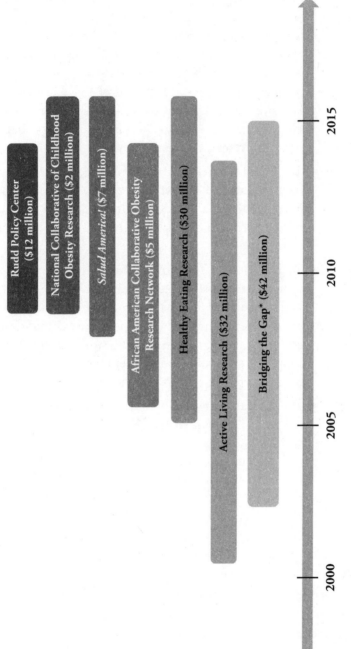

*Includes the dates and funding amount for childhood obesity–focused research only

## —⚯— Active Living Research

When James Sallis received his doctorate in clinical psychology in 1981, he approached the concept of active living as a behavioral psychologist would—with a focus on studying how to motivate individuals to exercise more. "That approach wasn't working at a scale that would make much of an impact in the grand scheme of things," says Sallis, who now runs Active Living Research out of the University of California, San Diego. But an editorial on the New Urbanism, an urban design movement popular in the 1980s, that promotes walkable neighborhoods, woke him to the idea of focusing on the built environment as a means of promoting not just walking but an overall active lifestyle. Today, his primary research interest is understanding policy and environmental influences on physical activity, nutrition, and obesity, particularly among children. "Childhood obesity is a wicked problem, one that requires the convergence of multiple approaches if we're going to ever solve it," he says.

To foster that convergence, Sallis and codirector Carmen Cutter have used Active Living Research as a platform to bring together investigators from such disciplines as urban planning, recreation, and transportation with those from the fields of public health, psychology, and sociology; the goal is to understand how people's interactions with their environment influence their desire and ability to be active outdoors. The thrust of the program, however, is employing research findings to effect policy. "A big part of what we do at Active Living Research now," Sallis says, "is to work on making the case for policymakers that their actions can have a positive impact on the health of the children in their communities."

A variety of projects funded by Active Living Research has shown, for example, that safe and attractive play spaces, such as school playgrounds and parks, are associated with higher activity levels in children and adolescents, which appears to translate into better weight control and even improved performance in school.

One study, conducted by Active Living Research grantee Myron Floyd, a professor in the Department of Parks, Recreation and Tourism Management at North Carolina State University, along with his colleagues in the Department of Sociology and Anthropology and the College of Design, examined how various aspects of park and playground design can increase or decrease activity among children and adolescents.[1] Floyd's work showed that children are more active when there are places for them to simply run around and be kids. Adolescents, however, are more active when there are features such as basketball courts, skate parks, and other areas that encourage social interaction while being active. That the parks were seen as being safe places was critical to overall activity, but for a somewhat unusual reason—parks seen as being less safe were associated with greater parental hovering, which had the effect of reducing activity levels.

Russell Lopez, an Active Living Research grantee at the Boston University School of Public Health, has shown that renovating dilapidated school playgrounds in Boston correlates with an increase in math test scores. Lopez completed a summary of all of the research showing the potential of safe, secure, and accessible playgrounds to increase children's physical activity.[2] Putting the results of this body of research into terms policymakers can understand, Lopez notes that policymakers and advocates can collaborate with schools to establish joint-use agreements that allow playing fields, playgrounds, and recreation centers to be used by community residents outside of school hours, and that city planners and local officials should work with community members to establish alternative policing strategies that can improve park safety and therefore increase activity levels among children and adolescents.

Translating research findings into policy recommendations is one side of the coin. The other, says program codirector Cutter, is to demonstrate that policies actually make a difference. "One of the areas that we and some of the other obesity-prevention programs have focused on is policy assessment," she explains. "If we can provide evidence that a local policy change has an impact on childhood obesity, then perhaps we can influence other communities to take action." For example, Active Living Research funded a study by Sara Benjamin Neelon, a child nutritionist and assistant professor in the Department of Community and Family Medicine at the Duke University Medical Center, to examine the effects of that policy change.[3] Based in part on the positive outcome of that study, she and her colleagues showed that few licensed child-care centers in North Carolina were doing all that they could to encourage healthy activity levels in children. As a result, North Carolina enacted a statewide policy that took effect in 2010 mandating that child-care settings increase daily levels of children's physical activity.

Jim Sallis says that the fact that policymakers are now willing to consider how the physical environment can affect children's health, and particularly childhood obesity, marks an important and promising change in thinking. "When Active Living Research was first funded," he says, "the entire emphasis in the obesity area was in the clinic and was focused on tackling this problem one person at a time, while today the major emphasis is on the environment and how we can shape that environment in ways that encourage active living and prevent obesity. I think the successes we're now seeing show that if we have the political will to enact smart policies, we can eliminate the problem of childhood obesity."

Aside from the reward of having a direct impact on childhood obesity, Sallis says one of the most satisfying aspects of his involvement with the program is the impact it has had on a generation of researchers. "Active Living Research has played the key role in creating an entire field of research that we hope will continue to have a positive impact on childhood obesity even after the program ends."

## —∿— Healthy Eating Research

Like Sallis, Mary Story, the director of Healthy Eating Research, came to the policy side of the child obesity battle as a refuge from the clinic; as a registered dietician she was counseling people who were trying to lose weight. "Working with individuals on weight control was very unsatisfying," she says, "because with a few exceptions, you don't really accomplish much." After completing her doctorate, Story got involved in designing community-based approaches to improving diet, focusing on children and adolescents in schools. The real turning point in her career came after a visit to a new school that had just opened in the Minneapolis suburb of Wayzata, where she noticed that there were thirty-five vending machines, "all of them filled with junk food." Dismayed, she went to the director of school nutrition for the State of Minnesota to ask for an explanation. The director responded with a simple question: "Why does it matter?"

Story didn't have an answer. "The fact of the matter was, there was no data to support the idea that getting rid of junk food at school had any impact on the overall health of kids; it was just an assumption that it would. I realized then that without hard data we would not be able to change the food environment in ways that would support healthy behavior."

With that impetus, Story conducted a small study on how price affected what students would eat at school. She convinced the food service directors at four schools to cut the price of fruits and vegetables in half, which led to a fourfold increase in the amount of fruits and vegetables the students ate. From there, she was off and running, and today—armed with reams of data, much of it generated by studies funded by Healthy Eating Research—Story is a regular in the offices of policymakers around the country.

Today, Healthy Eating Research issues competitive calls for research proposals, and it commissions small-scale research studies and analyses on topics addressing environmental factors leading to increased childhood obesity. Like Sallis, Story derives great satisfaction from mentoring and encouraging young researchers. She aims to help create a sustainable cadre of them, in part through the Foundation's New Connections grants to investigators representing populations and communities that are historically underrepresented in childhood obesity prevention research. "Healthy Eating Research has funded thirteen new investigators through New Connections," says Story, "and seeing these young researchers use these grants as springboards for their careers has been very rewarding." Story recently moved from the University of Minnesota, where Healthy Eating Research is still based, to Duke University.

Healthy Eating Research's effectiveness in improving food and nutrition policies, particularly those affecting schools and pre-schools, is due in part to the emphasis the program puts on smaller, shorter-duration grants. Running for a maximum of eighteen months and with up to $170,000 in funds, these grants are designed to inform timely and important policy debates and are modeled after a similar approach used by Active Living Research and the Robert Wood Johnson Foundation's Substance Abuse Policy Research Program. These "rapid-response" grants make up the entire Healthy Eating Research portfolio. "We're finding that these small, focused grants that answer specific, timely questions can produce big policy impacts," says Karen Kaphingst, the program's deputy director and one of Story's former students.

For example, Healthy Eating Research has funded several studies looking at the types of foods served at schools and preschools. One study, conducted by the Rudd Center, analyzed the foods served to children in preschool settings.[4] The Rudd Center turned those findings into a template specifying the foods children should receive, and that template has been adopted by Bright Horizons, a leading provider of preschool education and employer-sponsored child care. Another grant, to California Food Policy Advocates, examined what children ages two to five were eating and drinking in a variety of licensed child-care settings in California.[5] The findings provided a scientific basis that advocates were able to use to promote supportive legislation in all licensed child-care facilities. In 2010 California enacted legislation requiring early childhood programs to serve healthy beverages. "What's been fascinating to see," says Story, "is that when we then evaluated the impact of this legislation, we found that a large majority of licensed providers in California were eager to comply—but that they needed to be told how to do it. There was really no resistance among the providers."

On an even bigger stage, the body of evidence generated by Healthy Eating Research grantees provided a scientific under-pinning for the Healthy, Hunger-Free Kids Act of 2010, the legislation that authorizes funding and sets policy for the US Department of Agriculture's child nutrition programs. This legis-lation will lead to the first revamping of school meal programs in more than thirty years. One effect of the law will be to increase healthy food choices for students and reduce the availability of unhealthy snacks and sugar-sweetened beverages on school grounds that first drew Story's ire.

"That's particularly gratifying," she says, but now she has big-ger fish to fry. Asked what she would like to see happen next, she ticked off two top goals: ending all food marketing to children under seventeen and placing a tax on sugar-sweetened beverages. "The public health budget can't come close to competing with the marketing budget of the food industry," she says, "and we need to do something to level the playing field if we are serious about addressing the problem of childhood obesity."

## —⚬⚬— Bridging the Gap

Created in 1997 to assess the impact of policies, programs, and other environmental influences on adolescent alcohol, tobacco, and drug use, Bridging the Gap broadened its mandate in 2003 to include research on factors contributing to childhood obesity. Bridging the Gap is a joint initiative of two research projects: ImpacTeen, based at the Institute for Health Research and Policy at the University of Illinois at Chicago and overseen by codirector Frank Chaloupka; and Youth, Education & Society (YES), based at the Institute for Social Research at the University of Michigan and overseen by codirector Lloyd Johnston.

"Bridging the Gap is meant to be the research leg of the three-legged stool of research, action, and advocacy," explains Chaloupka, who came to the field of health economics when an economics class at John Carroll University, taught by one of the founders of the field, proved far more interesting than the organic chemistry class he was taking as a prerequisite for medical school. In fact, Chaloupka says one of the most enjoyable parts of his involvement with Bridging the Gap is being able to return the favor to the next generation of students—by showing them how interesting it can be to work in an interdisciplinary field studying how to influence such complicated and important behaviors.

One of his chief lieutenants in Bridging the Gap is Jamie Chriqui, a political scientist and health-policy researcher who first started analyzing the strength and comprehensiveness of state tobacco control laws for the National Cancer Institute in the late 1990s. "My *raison d'être* focuses on one issue—do laws and policies make a difference?" says Chriqui. "So what's been particularly exciting to me is not just the wonderful research we've been able to do, but more importantly that federal agencies have reached out to us to gain insights into what we've learned—particularly the US Department of Agriculture (USDA) as it developed the regulations required under the Healthy, Hunger-Free Kids Act of 2010." The result, she says, is that the program "has really helped bridge the gap in terms of the school food environment, providing the link between research findings and effective, life-changing policies." Chriqui is particularly pleased that kids coming through school today belong to the first generation to benefit from new public policies mandating that schools serve healthier food.

A major activity of Bridging the Gap is collecting data that Chriqui describes as "being both very detailed and nationwide in scope." For example, Bridging the Gap has been conducting a nationwide analysis of district wellness policies to evaluate how school districts are performing under a law enacted first by the federal government in 2004 and later strengthened by the Healthy, Hunger-Free Kids Act of 2010. Particularly relevant to the USDA's proposed rules for so-called competitive foods and beverages, meaning those sold at school outside of, and in competition with, the federally reimbursable meal programs, the analysis conducted by Bridging the Gap showed that competitive food and beverage provisions were the weakest pieces of district wellness plans.[6]

Under another data-collection effort, the Community Obesity Measures Project, data collectors go into 160 communities to observe consumer behavior in grocery stores, fast-food restaurants, parks, physical activity facilities, school grounds, and streets. The data are then compiled and made available to the research community. In one resulting study, Bridging the Gap team members found that the vast majority of fast-food restaurants promote their products to children through exterior signage, or community marketing, and that such marketing is more prevalent in low-income and African American and Latino neighborhoods.[7]

Another Bridging the Gap study looked at the promotion of unhealthy foods. Bridging the Gap investigator Lisa Powell collaborated with Jennifer Harris of the Rudd Center for Food Policy & Obesity and Tracy Fox of Food, Nutrition & Policy Consultants. Reexamining data underpinning a December 2012 report of the Federal Trade Commission that concluded that food and beverage companies spent nearly 20 percent less on marketing to children in 2009 than they did in 2006, the three researchers found that, in fact, the food and beverage industry still spends the bulk of its money to promote unhealthy products.[8] "Efforts by the food and beverage industry to self-regulate have proven ineffective at protecting children from exposure to advertisements for unhealthy products," the researchers concluded. "Existing industry-led standards and guidelines contain significant loopholes that allow continued marketing of products high in sugar, saturated fat, and sodium."

## —⚊— The Rudd Center for Food Policy & Obesity

That Healthy Eating Research's Mary Story wanted to see an end to all food marketing aimed at children under seventeen comes as no surprise, given the data generated by Yale University's Rudd Center for Food Policy & Obesity. Rudd's researchers focus much of their work on analyzing food marketing practices and economic conditions that create an environment placing the young and the poor at high risk of obesity. "When you look at the marketing practices of the major food and beverage companies and the fast-food industry," says Marlene Schwartz, who took over as director of the Rudd Center in July 2013 after founder Kelly Brownell left to become dean of the School of Public Health at Duke University, "they are really aimed at selling sugar-sweetened beverages, sugary cereals, and high-fat, high-salt snack food to children and adolescents. These companies have pledged to do better, and our studies show there have been some improvements. But they've been small and the pace of change is far too slow."

Schwartz, a former clinical psychologist who, like Story, came to the public policy arena after becoming disheartened by working with individuals on weight control and obesity, is motivated by the David and Goliath aspect of countering the impact of multibillion-dollar marketing budgets of the fast-food and food and beverage industries. "The fast-food industry spent $4.6 billion dollars on advertising in 2012," she says. "McDonald's alone spent 2.7 times as much to advertise its products as all fruit, vegetable, bottled water, and milk advertisers combined."

Rudd Center research found that in 2012, US preschoolers viewed an average of 2.8 fast-food ads on television every day; children aged six to eleven viewed 3.2 ads per day; and teens viewed 4.8 ads per day. African American children and adolescents saw at least 50 percent more such ads than their white peers. "And those figures don't count all of the advertising that children and adolescents are exposed to on the Internet and other new media," says Schwartz.

A similar situation exists concerning unhealthy snacks and sugar-sweetened beverages. A recent study from the Rudd Center showed that professional athletes, who serve as particularly effective marketing tools to adolescents, overwhelmingly endorse beverages that get all of their calories from added sugars.[9] As part of its efforts to counter these practices, the Rudd Center encourages food companies to improve their marketing practices and their products, and it monitors the extent to which those companies are honoring their pledges.

Research by the Rudd Center investigators also showed that while most fast-food restaurants have made positive changes in kids' meals between 2010 and 2013, the meals are still too high in calories, saturated fat, sugar, and sodium. "Finding the healthy options for kids at a fast-food restaurant is like finding a needle in a haystack," says Rudd researcher Jennifer Harris, "and even then, you have to specifically ask for them."

The Rudd Center's investigators conducted a two-part analysis of fast-food nutrition and marketing. First, they looked at data produced during a study they conducted in 2010—four years after the food industry pledged to self-regulate its advertising to children and adolescents—and then they did a follow-up analysis in 2012. Known as Fast Food F.A.C.T.S. (Food Advertising to Children and Teens Score), Cereal F.A.C.T.S., and Sugary Drinks F.A.C.T.S., these surveys provide a wealth of information for food advocates and consumers across the nation and create a foundation for pressuring the fast-food industry to change its practices.

"The data in the Fast Food F.A.C.T.S. survey, as well as the others that the Rudd Center conducts on other aspects of food industry practices, show clearly that the food and beverage companies are taking a page from the tobacco industry playbook," says Kelly Brownell, who, during his years as director of the Rudd Center, largely abandoned the idea of trying to play nice with the food industry; instead, he became one of its most outspoken and visible critics.

"These companies will pledge to make changes, but they do it very slowly if at all," he says. "They will continue to deny that their products have any relationship to adverse health effects—in spite of mounting evidence that the opposite is true. They use pricing and marketing to push their products to the most vulnerable populations. Given all that, if we as a nation really want to address the problem of childhood obesity, we need to stop trying to be reasonable with industry because it will not work. Instead, we need to get out the bludgeon of legislation that restricts marketing to children and taxes on sugar-sweetened beverages." Brownell is critical of the Robert Wood Johnson Foundation for shying away from taking this more adversarial approach toward the fast-food and food and beverage industries.

### —ᗯ— Salud America! The Robert Wood Johnson Foundation Research Network to Prevent Obesity Among Latino Children

Salud America! director Amelie Ramirez is particularly alarmed by the fact that more than 39 percent of Latino children ages two to nineteen are overweight or obese, compared to almost 32 percent of all US children. "When you consider that Latino children comprise 22 percent of all US youth and represent the largest and youngest minority group in the nation," she says, "the high prevalence of obesity in Latino children is a time bomb that could have severe consequences for the nation as a whole."

With a master's of public health in health services administration and a doctorate that focused on the use of public health approaches and community-based prevention to address complex unhealthy behaviors, Ramirez has spent her professional career documenting and addressing health disparities among minority communities. Part of this effort has involved creating a network of researchers and community advocates with expertise in the unique cultural and socioeconomic factors at work in

Latino communities. Initially, Ramirez's focus was on creating such a network to reach Latina women with breast cancer; now, thanks to Robert Wood Johnson Foundation funding for Salud America!, she and her colleagues are taking on the problem of addressing the obesity epidemic affecting Latino children.

Toward that end, Salud America! is an online national network of more than three thousand experts, community leaders, and advocates who work together to identify high-priority issues and then conduct the research needed to address those issues. More than twenty Salud America! grants have gone to strengthen the network. The grants have been directed at funding network investigators, many of whom are Latino, who had not worked in childhood obesity prevention. Many subsequently received funding from the National Institutes of Health and other sources.

Salud America! concentrates its research funding in six areas: healthier school snacks, better food in the neighborhood, active spaces, active play, healthier marketing, and sugary drinks. One study, led by Carmen Nevarez of the Public Health Institute, evaluated the impact of a voluntary menu-labeling program called *La Salud Tiene Sabor*, in heavily Latino South Los Angeles.[10] The evaluation team found that nearly two-thirds of restaurant patrons saw the nutritional information provided by the participating restaurants, and that nearly half of these said it influenced their purchase choices. The researchers also found that some restaurant owners changed their own eating behaviors because of the program and now promote healthy eating choices to their customers. Finally, the majority of restaurant owners surveyed reported no notable changes in costs and profits from the program and said that they would recommend it to other small, independent restaurant owners.

Another research project funded by Salud America! is called *Esto es Mejor:* Improving Food Purchasing Selection among Low-Income, Spanish-Speaking Latinos through Social Marketing Messages. This program examined how simplified nutritional information online could be used to improve food literacy and increase healthy eating among low-income Spanish-speaking Latinos.[11]

The Salud America! network includes community leaders and advocates who can spread the word locally. "One of the real strengths of the Salud America! network," says Kipling "Kip" Gallion, Salud America!'s deputy director, "is that it provides a steady stream of examples of successful efforts to counter negative influences and make progress in fighting childhood obesity. We can then feed these examples back to the network as a whole." Gallion, whose expertise lies in health communications, has known Ramirez since the early 1980s, when they were both students of Alfred McAlister, a pioneer in tobacco control research at the University of Texas School of Public Health in Houston. Ramirez and Gallion were learning the value of public health approaches to address health disparities.

Today, much of Salud America!'s program staff, which is based at the University of Texas Health Science Center in San Antonio, works at sharing success stories and helpful resources for dissemination via the program's Web site. One of the program's major efforts has been preparing packages of research reviews, issues briefs, and videos in Spanish and English, and summary infographics for each of the program's six areas of emphasis for reversing Latino childhood obesity. Each of these packages distills five-plus years of research into materials for use by community leaders and advocates.

The program also asks community members to share their success stories in these six areas via the Web site. Salud America! staff members then conduct interviews, write stories, and film those stories to create professional-quality videos for dissemination to a national audience. One story, for example, tells of Caesar Valdillez's efforts to help his heavily Latino neighborhood in San Antonio establish a city-supported community garden—a means of providing access to fresh vegetables in an area where the only nearby source of groceries is convenience stores. The video that the Salud America! staff produced not only tells a compelling story, but also provides nuts-and-bolts details that other communities can now use to take action.

## —∿— The African American Collaborative Obesity Research Network (AACORN)

Like Salud America!'s Amelie Ramirez, AACORN's Shiriki Kumanyika is building a community of researchers, in this case one comprising investigators with grounding in African American life experiences and obesity-related scientific expertise. "There are a great many cultural issues in the African American community related to food and weight that make it a politically difficult area to work in," says Kumanyika, who has a Master's in public health and a PhD in nutrition and whose academic career at the University of Pennsylvania School of Medicine has focused on public health and nutrition issues. "By putting together a network of researchers who are well-versed in the social and cultural aspects of the African American community, we have been able to emphasize the point that our children are an intimate part of our community and that the community needs to make changes to support our children's overall health as a means of fighting obesity."

A turning point in this effort occurred in 2004, she says, when this network of researchers met for an entire day of discussion and debate as part of AACORN's first national workshop. Looking at the evidence from a wide range of fields, the workshop participants concluded that focusing on body weight was not the way to solve the childhood obesity problem in African American communities. Instead, the emphasis should be placed on healthy behavior as a whole.

In 2007, AACORN published this new obesity paradigm and called for a broader interdisciplinary and contextualized approach to designing interventions on eating, physical activity, and weight, with particular reference to African Americans. The paradigm suggests that weight-control interventions must be informed by a broader knowledge base about life in African American communities; it also must be framed more holistically to consider other relevant social and health priorities and adaptations to adverse life circumstances.[12]

Since that workshop, AACORN's focus has been to build on this consensus and to take aim at a two-pronged problem that Kumanyika says is particularly pernicious in the African American community—price inequality between healthy and unhealthy food combined with culturally targeted marketing of unhealthy food and beverages. "I think the key issue here is to pull the right levers so that communities see this as a social justice issue and that they have the ability to demand better treatment from the food industry," says Kumanyika.

As one example, AACORN-funded investigators have been working with community leaders in Little Rock, Arkansas, to involve both consumers and retailers in an effort to improve health food availability and reduce in-store marketing of unhealthy foods. Using data showing that this can be a win-win situation for all parties, this effort is gaining traction there and is starting to make a positive impact. "This kind of proof-of-principle demonstration is what we're focused on now so that we can convince members of the community that they can have an impact and need to be involved," she says.

Another AACORN study looked at how fast-food marketing to parents influences their children's consumption of fast food. The investigators surveyed parents of children receiving care at federally funded community health centers on the East Coast and in Puerto Rico—children at high risk of obesity and related health problems. The results of the survey showed that children's fast-food consumption was directly associated with parental exposure to fast-food marketing.[13]

## —∿— Conclusion: An Eye to the Future

The portfolio of childhood obesity research programs supported by the Robert Wood Johnson Foundation had a triple purpose: first, to produce a body of research that would provide a scientific base for policy change; second, to create a network of childhood obesity researchers; and third, to strengthen the new field of childhood obesity research.

As this chapter has illustrated, at least some Foundation-funded research did provide a scientific grounding for public policies aimed at reducing childhood obesity. Research in North Carolina funded under Active Living Research led to a statewide change that increased physical activity in child-care centers. Research supported by Bridging the Gap was used by the USDA in formulating regulations. Research financed under Healthy Eating Research provided an underpinning for improved nutrition in pre-kindergarten settings. Well-publicized research by the Rudd Center has put pressure on fast-food chains to sell healthier food. In addition, says Foundation senior vice president Jim Marks, research funded by the Robert Wood Johnson Foundation provided an underpinning for the Institute of Medicine's recommendations on reducing childhood obesity.

Although the Robert Wood Johnson Foundation wasn't the only organization funding research into nonbiological factors that contribute to the childhood obesity epidemic, the Foundation's obesity research efforts undoubtedly strengthened the field. "There were individuals doing research in the field before the Robert Wood Johnson Foundation," says Active Living Research's Jim Sallis, "but what the program really did was create opportunities for raising an entire generation of researchers interested in childhood obesity. Equally important, it brought in researchers from a wide range of fields who didn't know that the work they were doing was relevant to childhood obesity. The effect of bringing in these different perspectives is that we now have a vibrant, multidisciplinary field that is not only producing results that are interesting, but results that are usable by communities and that are influencing policy." These researchers now communicate with each other through networks developed under AACORN, Salud America!, and the other research programs supported by the Foundation.

The Foundation is now trying to solidify the gains made in reducing childhood obesity by moving more toward demonstration projects and creating policy and advocacy briefs. "The idea," says childhood obesity team leader Dwayne Proctor, "is that we now want to start translating all of this great research into action." As one example, in 2013, the Foundation agreed to co-fund an $8 million collaboration with the American Heart Association to create and manage an advocacy initiative focused on changing local, state, and federal policies to help children and adolescents eat healthier foods and be more active.

Still, with uncertainty about the level of federal funding for research on childhood obesity, researchers in the field are nervous. "The field is just reaching critical mass," says Healthy Eating Research's Mary Story, "and at a time when federal research funds are shrinking, any shift in the Foundation's support could hamper our efforts—just at the point where we've generated a significant body of research to support steps needed to make a major impact on childhood obesity." This is a feeling voiced repeatedly by researchers involved in the Foundation's childhood obesity initiative.

An initiative now its fifth year—the National Collaborative on Childhood Obesity Research—offers one way of continuing support. Begun in 2008, the collaborative is a joint effort of the Robert Wood Johnson Foundation, the Centers for Disease Control and Prevention, the USDA, and the National Institutes of Health. Its research into policy and environmental interventions to reduce obesity in children and adolescents from low-income and minority families is particularly timely.

And as long as childhood obesity remains a serious health concern in the United States, research on it will continue. As the Foundation's Dwayne Proctor observes, the Robert Wood Johnson Foundation may shift its focus in terms of the type of research it funds, but its commitment to research is unwavering. "Yes, we're moving more towards demonstration projects and creating policy and advocacy briefs," he says, "but the Foundation always works from an evidence base and we're still going to need research to bolster what we're doing in these new areas related to childhood obesity."

## Notes

1. M. F. Floyd, et al., "Park-Based Activity Among Children and Adolescents," *American Journal of Preventive Medicine* 41, no. 3 (2011): 258–65.

2. R. Lopez, "The Potential of Safe, Secure and Accessible Playgrounds to Increase Children's Physical Activity. Policy Brief for Active Living Research," 2011, http://activelivingresearch.org/sites/default/files/ALR_Brief_SafePlaygrounds_0.pdf. Accessed 5/22/2014.

3. A. L. Cradock, et al., "A Review of State Regulations to Promote Physical Activity and Safety on Playgrounds in Child Care Centers and Family Child Care Homes," *Journal of Physical Activity & Health* 7, Suppl. 1 (2010): S108–19.

4. M. L. O'Connell, et al., "Repeated Exposure in a Natural Setting: A Preschool Intervention to Increase Vegetable Consumption," *Journal of the Academy of Nutrition and Dietetics* 112, no. 2 (2012): 230-34.

5. K. Hecht, et al., "Nutrition and Physical Activity Environments in Licensed Child Care: A Statewide Assessment of California," A Report for Health Eating Research, 2009, http://cfpa.net/ChildNutrition/ChildCare/CFPAPublications/RWJF-StatewideChildCareAssessment-2009.pdf. Accessed 5/22/2014.

6. L. M. Schneider, et al., "The Extent to Which School District Competitive Food and Beverage Policies Align with the 2010 Dietary Guidelines for Americans: Implications for Federal Regulations," *Journal of the Academy of Nutrition and Dietetics* 112, no. 6 (2012): 892–96.

7. L. M. Powell, et al., *Exterior Marketing Practices of Fast-Food Restaurants*—A BTG Research Brief. Chicago: Bridging the Gap Program, Health Policy Center, Institute for Health Research and Policy, University of Illinois at Chicago, 2012, http://www.bridgingthegapresearch.org/_asset/2jc2wr/btg_fast_food_pricing_032012.pdf. Accessed 5/22/2014.

8. L. M. Powell, et al., "Food Marketing Expenditures Aimed at Youth: Putting the Numbers in Context," *American Journal of Preventive Medicine* 45, no. 4 (2013): 453–61.

9. M. A. Bragg, et al., "Athlete Endorsements in Food Marketing," *Pediatrics* 132, no. 5 (2013): 805–10.

10. C. R. Navarez, et al., "*Salud Tiene Sabor*: A Model for Healthier Restaurants in a Latino Community," *American Journal of Preventive Medicine* 44, 3S3 (2013): S186–92.

11. D. E. Cortés, "Improving Food Purchasing Selection among Low-Income Spanish-Speaking Latinos," Research Brief for *Salud America!*, 2011, https://salud-america.org/sites/salud-america/files/grantee-research /Cortes2011-research-brief_0.pdf. Accessed 5/22/2014.

12. S. K. Kumanyika, et al., "Expanding the Obesity Research Paradigm to Reach African American Communities," *Preventing Chronic Disease* 4, no. 4: [A112], http://www.cdc.gov/pcd/issues/2007/oct/07_0067.htm. Accessed 2/1/2014.

13. S. A. Grier, et al., "Fast-Food Marketing and Children's Fast-Food Consumption: Exploring Parents' Influences in an Ethnically Diverse Sample," *Journal of Public Policy & Marketing* 26, no 2 (2007): 221–35.

# The Robert Wood Johnson Foundation's Programs to Improve the Built Environment

*Will Bunch*

## Introduction

The founders of the Robert Wood Johnson Foundation saw its purpose as addressing issues of medical care in the United States; this perspective lasted two decades. The major programs initiated in the 1970s aimed at increasing access to medical care, especially outpatient care. Even during the 1980s, when the Foundation broadened its concerns to include long-term care, the behaviors that spread AIDS, and supportive housing, the staff and Board continued to think of the Foundation as a medical-care philanthropy. Nonetheless, according to Alan Cohen, a former Foundation vice president for research and evaluation, staff members in the mid- to late 1980s began to recognize the relationship between social problems and health.

In the 1990s, under the leadership of Steven Schroeder, the Foundation conducted a major campaign against the harms of tobacco, the leading preventable cause of death. The tobacco programming, which aimed at changing behavior (reducing smoking), broadened the Foundation's focus and implicitly put it in the business of improving health. Near the end of his presidency,

Schroeder made the expanded focus explicit by making health an equal partner to health care.[1]

In addition to the efforts to discourage smoking under Schroeder's presidency, the Foundation also tried to influence other unhealthy behaviors, such as alcohol and drug abuse and lack of exercise. Beginning around 2000, the Foundation began exploring ways to increase the opportunity for physical activity by improving the built environment—that is, by making it easier for residents of communities to walk, run, or bicycle—through a series of Active Living programs.[2]

With the priority given to reducing childhood obesity under Risa Lavizzo-Mourey's presidency, the early 2000s efforts to make communities friendlier to bikers, runners, and walkers were greatly amplified. As Will Bunch reports in this chapter, the Foundation funded major programs designed to improve nutrition and physical activity. In addition, the Foundation began to explore broader approaches to making communities healthier, even working with the Federal Reserve Board to examine how community development influences health.

The transformation of the Foundation from a philanthropy focused on medical care to one focused on health was completed in 2014 when, under Lavizzo-Mourey's leadership, the Foundation adopted a new vision: to advance a culture of health that will enable everyone in our diverse society to lead healthy lives. Improving the built environment is one of the ways of producing a culture of health, and, as Bunch writes, it is an area in which the Foundation has had considerable experience. Bunch is an award-winning journalist with the *Philadelphia Daily News*. He has written frequently for the *Anthology*, most recently contributing a chapter on The Food Trust for Volume XV.

## Notes

1. J. M. McGinnis and S. A. Schroeder, "Expanding the Focus of the Robert Wood Johnson Foundation: Health as an Equal Partner to Health Care," in S. L. Isaacs and J. R. Knickman (eds), *To Improve Health and Health Care: The Robert Wood Johnson Foundation Anthology 2001* (San Francisco: Jossey-Bass, 2001).
2. S. McGrath, "The Active Living Programs," in S. L. Isaacs and D. C. Colby (eds), *To Improve Health and Health Care: The Robert Wood Johnson Foundation Anthology* Vol. XI (San Francisco: Jossey-Bass, 2007).

—⁓— In popular culture, the years immediately following World War II in America have been branded "the baby boom" era, as millions of young veterans returned home to start families. But in fact, the rising national birth rate actually paled in those years compared to the explosion in auto registrations; while there were just twenty-six million cars on the road at war's end, by the 1950s that number had skyrocketed to forty million.

In June 1956, President Dwight Eisenhower signed the law that created the United States interstate highway system. Planners like New York's Robert Moses increased the pace of freeway construction to accommodate the new cars and drivers. The iconic image from that time is the aerial shot of brand new suburbs such as Long Island's Levittown, a mosaic of twisting residential streets and cul-de-sacs as far as the eye can see, and on those streets a numbing pattern of repeated Cape Cod–style homes, each with a driveway of glistening asphalt. It took a perfect storm of factors to spark the rapid suburbanization of America, including federally subsidized college education and mortgages for returning G.I.s, as well as their desire to raise their kids amid fresh-mown lawns. But the automobile made it go.

It did not take long for a backlash to emerge. In 1961, the social critic and writer Jane Jacobs published *The Death and Life of Great American Cities*, which argued that most urban renewal plans caused inadvertent harm by robbing city neighborhoods of the traits that made them most livable: a mixture of uses and types of architecture that would connect people from different walks of life at all times of the day, creating a thriving urban village like Manhattan's Greenwich Village, where Jacobs then lived.

The broader debate that Jacobs helped to trigger gradually led to such urban planning movements as the New Urbanism, which took root in the 1980s and 1990s as a counterweight to the prevailing suburban car culture; it emphasized either newly built or revitalized existing neighborhoods with a mix of homes, stores, and offices, walkable streets, and easy access to mass transit. Many people saw New Urbanism as a tool for implementing so-called Smart Growth, a broader strategy for reducing sprawl.

Public health experts began to enter the debate over suburban sprawl, with good reason. By the late 1990s, there was growing evidence that the amount of time Americans were spending on the road—kids taking a bus to school instead of walking or bicycling, their parents driving to a supermarket instead of walking to a corner market—was making them less physically fit and even obese. City planners and health advocates concluded that making changes in what they called the built environment—engineering new opportunities to walk or bike—would improve not just the social well-being of a community, but also its physical fitness.

Beginning in 1999, the Robert Wood Johnson Foundation developed an interest in the built environment, and it began to support a series of initiatives throughout the nation. More than a dozen years later, the first generation of built environment projects—including those supported by the Foundation through such flagship programs as Active Living By Design, Healthy Kids, Healthy Communities, and a half-dozen smaller efforts—has brought mixed-to-positive results in rolling back an entrenched car culture. Overall, experts agree that the pioneering push for more walking and cycling opportunities has generated enough success stories that many cities and towns have moved toward the next phase, one that could be called built environment 2.0.

In the mid-2010s, the generation of urban planners who cut their teeth advocating for bike lanes and crosswalks are increasingly in positions of local power, and they've been using their newfound political clout to expand the breadth of a built environment agenda. For example:

  ■ A growing number of city and metropolitan governing and planning bodies are making sidewalks and other pedestrian-friendly upgrades a mandatory element of revised zoning codes for developers and for renovation projects, and are requiring lanes for cyclists when roads are repaved or widened.

- In the second generation of projects, advocates for a more active lifestyle are more focused than before on the problem of equity—that is, making sure that infrastructure improvements and community programs reach the poorest neighborhoods and communities, where research has shown that rates of obesity and related diseases tend to be higher.

- Particularly in urban centers, active living programs have increasingly merged with newer efforts to improve what some advocates now call "the food environment," involving community gardens or larger urban farms that produce fresh produce for so-called "food deserts," as well as through siting new supermarkets or farmers' markets so that residents without access to cars can pick up healthier foods within walking distance of home.

- Growing alarm over the health and fitness of young people—fueled by findings that the number of children who became dangerously overweight doubled between the early 1980s and 2000—has led to a shift in focus on more programs that target youth at risk for obesity. Partly because of the new focus, active living programs that were once largely the province of urban planners and transportation engineers are now increasingly run out of health departments.

## —∞— A Suite of Programs to Improve the Built Environment

In 2001, the Robert Wood Johnson Foundation announced the creation of a portfolio of six closely related projects and a financial commitment of $56 million, aimed at different aspects of advancing the same goal: changing the physical environment of communities so that their residents could adopt a healthier lifestyle by increased walking, biking, and other forms of physical activity. Indeed, when a handful of Foundation program officers and public health experts from the Centers for Disease Control and Prevention and others began discussing such a campaign near the end of the 1990s, participants said they were not even sure what to call it. "We brought in the term 'active living,' a term being used in Australia and in Canada," says Kate Kraft, a former program officer at the Foundation who was a chief architect in developing the initial portfolio, "and we looked at how to reengineer back into our lives all the things that had been engineered out of our lives, such as walking to school or to a neighborhood grocery store."

The participants in planning the active living programs shared several beliefs. One was that a direct connection existed between the nation's post–World War II suburban-oriented car culture, with its rising rates of physical inactivity among both adults and children, and a higher incidence of heart disease, diabetes, and other ailments. The second shared belief was that advertising-oriented campaigns that simply encouraged viewers to hit the gym or go for a long walk were not having much impact, especially as more and more Americans moved to exurban communities lacking such basic amenities for exercising as parks, or even sidewalks. The participants also believed that they would need to change not only the habits of car-owning citizens, but also the entrenched mindset of politicians, public agencies, and career transportation planners.

### Active Living By Design

The most visible of the new programs was Active Living By Design, which initially awarded approximately $200,000 apiece to twenty-five localities for pilot projects, most involving physical improvements to the built environment; the competition sparked wide national interest, attracting more than nine hundred applications.

Headquartered in the University of North Carolina Gillings School of Global Public Health at Chapel Hill, Active Living By Design looked to diversify its pilot projects so that researchers, future funders, and communities would get the best sense of what worked in promoting physical activity. Some of the programs supported seemingly modest efforts such as walking clubs or Safe Routes to School. Other, more ambitious efforts promoted high-profile projects like biking or walking trails, or policy changes such as zoning codes to require sidewalks in new developments.

### Active Living Research

Headed by James Sallis, Distinguished Professor of Family and Preventive Medicine at the University of California, San Diego, who has been studying the link between physical inactivity and health outcomes since the 1980s, Active Living Research was established to finance research projects on the built environment. The goal was to identify what types of projects in this brand-new strategy were successful and which ones faltered—and why.

Over its decade of existence, Active Living Research has funded more than two hundred research projects and has made its findings widely accessible to health policy officials eager to know the best built environment practices to promote healthy living. Sallis is passionate in describing the goal of fostering connections between fields that don't always communicate well. "We must deepen the collaboration between public health and all other relevant sectors," he says. "We want to move toward health in all policies. Every sector needs to think about how they are contributing to health, in positive and negative ways."

### Other Active Living Programs

The first wave of Foundation-backed programs also included a batch of smaller, focused campaigns with similar goals of sharing information about the built environment and creating evangelists for the concept. These included Active Living Leadership, later renamed Leadership for Healthy Communities, a policy arm that offered advice and technical support to civic leaders; two programs, the Active Living Network and the Active Living Resource Center, that offered information and technical research to professionals and activists; and a program called Active for Life, established to encourage exercise among adults over age fifty.

### The Convergence Partnership

In the fall of 2005, the Foundation joined with Kaiser Permanente, The California Endowment, the W. K. Kellogg Foundation, Nemours, and, later, with other leading philanthropies to support the Healthy Eating/Active Living Convergence Partnership; it is now known simply as the Convergence Partnership. The effort came about because a number of philanthropies began focusing on built environment projects at the same time, and they wanted to coordinate their efforts.

John Govea, the Foundation's senior program officer for the Convergence Partnership, says the project provides a way for leading nonprofits that tend to specialize in diverse areas (for example, The Kresge Foundation, which is strong in transportation and infrastructure) to collaborate on experimental healthy living ideas that transcend their traditional silos. "What the Convergence Partnership brings," says Govea, "is that the partners all tend to look at things differently."

### The Healthy Kids, Healthy Communities Program

The Healthy Kids, Healthy Communities Program, which was run from the same office at the University of North Carolina at Chapel Hill that managed Active Living By Design, funded dozens of small-scale, collaborative projects across the country designed to increase physical activity and access to healthy food. Although some of these projects continued the work of Active Living By

Design in building and promoting new venues for bicycling or walking, others focused on community food issues such as supermarket siting. Some Healthy Kids, Healthy Communities projects targeted the exercise needs of children in new ways, such as "shared use" agreements to make school playing fields available to young people who are not students there.

### County Health Rankings & Roadmaps

In January 2009, the Foundation announced a $4.9 million grant to the University of Wisconsin Population Health Institute with the goal of taking nationwide a project that the Institute had initially launched on a statewide basis six years earlier—to map health-related behaviors and amenities on a county-by-county basis. The project, now known as County Health Rankings & Roadmaps, aims to provide useful data to community leaders, as well as to show that an array of factors—including opportunities for physical activity in the built environment—can affect health outcomes.

"We want people to learn that there's a lot more to health than health care," says Bridget Booske Catlin, the senior scientist at the Wisconsin Institute who is director of the program. "One of the messages is to have more people talking about the social determinants of health, and using things like the built environment to improve health. We need to look outside of the walls of the doctor's office."

Beginning in 2010, County Health Rankings & Roadmaps has released annual surveys, using within-state comparisons to show where counties stand on a broad array of factors, including air and water pollution, percentage of high school graduates, children living in single-parent households, rates of alcohol abuse, and much more. Increasingly, says Catlin, the focus has turned to the Roadmaps aspect of the program—a tool developed to help area politicians, planners, philanthropies, educators, and activists translate the rankings into policies that will promote better health. The program, which was renewed in 2014, has become a centerpiece in the Foundation's effort to advance a culture of health.

## —⚬— A Tale of Three Cities

Three widely divergent cities, whose stories are told in detail below, illustrate the variety of approaches taken to increase the opportunities for physical activity. They are Buffalo, New York; Nashville, Tennessee; and Louisville, Kentucky.

### Buffalo, New York

One of the more than nine hundred cities that competed for the first round of Active Living By Design grants more than a decade ago was Buffalo, the upstate New York outpost that today is known for its "lake effect" snow, its zesty chicken wings, and its vacant buildings; at the height of the Industrial Revolution, however, Buffalo was famed for its splendid system of parks and grand boulevards.

Buffalo's initial application for a Foundation grant was unique in that it came not from a public agency, but rather from the city's dynamic and fastest-growing nongovernmental employer, Buffalo Niagara Medical Campus (BNMC). Buffalo's built environment program started small, by focusing on an underdeveloped neighborhood on the outskirts of downtown. Today, it's hailed by local activists for inspiring a civic renaissance in community gardens and bicycling.

The view from a large picture window on the third floor of Buffalo's Innovation Center, where the community development arm of the medical center, BNMC, Inc., has its office, offers a diorama of how a once-faceless pedestrian-unfriendly one-way street is becoming a haven for walkers and cyclists. On the opposite side of Ellicott Street, being reengineered from one-way to two-way to slow down traffic, a wide ribbon of ground between the roadway and a grim surface parking lot is well on the way to becoming Elli-cott Park. Young trees are ringed by artfully designed and inviting new park benches and low-level lighting. Twenty or so gleaming new bicycles, GPS-equipped, sit in stands waiting for BNMC staff or visitors to share, while, behind an orange construction fence on the near side of the street, workers are busy creating a swath of greenway that will stretch for more than a half mile, all the way to a stop on Buffalo's subway line. Beyond the parking lot rise a church spire and the roofs of a public housing project that mark the city's historically poor neighborhood called "the Fruit Belt." BNMC officials are optimistic that Ellicott Park will offer not just recreation but also a pathway to jobs, as the medical center con-tinues its plan to add five thousand new workers over the next few years.

Michael Ball was director of campus planning for the medical center when it created BNMC, Inc., at the dawn of the 2000s. Ball says the center's officials saw a remarkable opportunity when they applied for an Active Living By Design grant in 2003. Not only was the program a way for BNMC to transform what had been an uninviting no man's land around its main downtown campus; it could also become a mechanism for forging a new working rela-tionship with the lower-income, predominantly black residents and leaders of the Fruit Belt and Allentown neighborhoods. These people had come to distrust the hospital during its earlier growth spurts. "They didn't trust the institutional leadership," says Ball, "because they'd seen the neighborhood erode. But the neighbors told us that could change if we could get things done—they'd never even been able to get the streetlights to work."

So the medical center began working with the neighborhood's leaders and the City of Buffalo on simple issues, such as the bro-ken streetlighting; they located new crosswalks where kids walk to school; and they created a small new park on the edge of the Fruit Belt near the medical campus. By starting small, Buffalo's Active

Living pilot project not only improved BNMC's immediate surroundings; it also helped foster a wider sense that Smart Growth should be an integral part of the city's rebirth.

Despite jokes about snowy winter weather and the steady decline of its traditional smokestack industries, Buffalo retains the core of its acclaimed greenways, created by the legendary late-nineteenth-century park planner Frederick Law Olmsted. Also remaining are stately historic mansions evoking a bygone era, now often sitting among abandoned lots. By the 2000s, such assets began to attract New Urbanism advocates to Buffalo—people willing to trade a few months of bone-chilling winter for a climate of networking, idea sharing, and optimism about Smart Growth in a surprising city.

A nonprofit initially called Green Options Buffalo was formed; it advocated adding bike lanes whenever major city streets were repaved, launched a bicycle-recycling program for Buffalo youth, and successfully lobbied for a city ordinance requiring pedestrian-friendly "complete streets" (that is, streets that keep *all users* in mind, including bicyclists, public transportation vehicles and riders, and pedestrians) to accompany any reconstruction project.

Today, activist Justin Booth is the public—and towering—face of how Buffalo transformed its built environment. The six-foot nine-inch Brooklyn native came to play basketball at Buffalo State College, then married a hometown woman and never left. Now thirty-five, he's the executive director of GObike Buffalo, the successor to Green Options Buffalo; GObike Buffalo is housed on the BNMC campus.

On a steely-gray, rainy morning in late November, Booth steps outside a crowded coffee shop in the heart of the downtown Delaware Avenue commercial corridor, where more than a mile of new bike lanes were added in 2013; even he is surprised to see a half-dozen bicycles parked in a rack in such bad weather. "There is a lot of redevelopment along Delaware Avenue," Booth says, "so it's great to see the city do this along such a high-traffic street.

There haven't been any major complaints about Delaware Avenue—the only thing we hear is, 'Why hasn't this happened to my street?'"

It might happen soon. Of Buffalo's roughly forty miles of bike lanes, says Booth, about thirty miles have been created in the last three years. In 2012, the League of American Bicyclists sifted through US Census Bureau data to determine that Buffalo is the sixth fastest-growing city of bicycle commuting in the nation. On a tour of the city, Booth proudly shows off a small but significant symbol of that progress: the city's first traffic signal just for cyclists. It's on Linwood Avenue, a handsome residential street recently converted to one-way auto traffic to make room for bikes.

But promoting cycling is not Booth's only contribution to a healthier environment in Buffalo. In the once-vacant lot next to his sturdy red-brick, turn-of-the-century home just east of the downtown core, Booth and his wife have worked with their neighbors to create a lush community garden where a crushed stone walkway loops past sunflower plants and willow trees. The site is attractive, but not unique—the nonprofit Grassroots Gardens of Buffalo has watched roughly seventy such gardens take root across the city, many amid architectural gems on the city's west side.

The flourishing community garden culture in Buffalo is another tangible symbol of the newer phase of the built environment movement, which is increasingly focused on the food environment. The goal is to spotlight access to fruits and vegetables and other healthy foods, some grown locally in gardens or on an increasing number of urban farms on larger abandoned tracts. Another priority is finding locations for, and supporting construction of, small grocery stores or supermarkets that sell produce, especially in urban locations that can be reached on foot. When the Robert Wood Johnson Foundation established the Healthy Kids, Healthy Communities program in 2007, Buffalo was one of eight cities from the original Active Living By Design project to win a grant from the new effort.

"We recognized that we were in the midst of a food desert, that kids in the Fruit Belt simply did not have healthy food options," says Samina Raja, an associate professor in the School of Architecture and Planning at the University at Buffalo, State University of New York. Raja, who has partnered with the Healthy Kids, Healthy Communities program, was an early proponent of urban gardens; she also worked with local activist Diane Picard to introduce and promote healthier foods in a neighborhood middle school on an eighteen-month, $50,000 Robert Wood Johnson grant under the Active Living By Design program.

Under Healthy Kids, Healthy Communities, Raja and other activists have been working on a wide array of projects: some are narrow in scope—for example, Raja has advised a new youth advisory board in the Buffalo school district that encourages students to advocate for healthier food and wellness programs—and others broad and bold, most notably the adoption of a new "green code" to replace the city's outdated zoning code. The green code encourages, and often mandates, sidewalks or complete streets; it also recognizes the value of assets like community gardens.

Perhaps most critically, some New Urbanism advocates have moved up the ladder as local decision makers—for instance, Michael Ball, the former director of campus planning for the medical center, is now a state official in his role as a deputy director of Empire State Development. "I think," says Raja, "that we learned how to get things done in this city."

### Nashville, Tennessee

Like many American cities, Nashville began its push to become a more active city organically. Back in the late 1990s, Bill Purcell was elected mayor. This so-called "neighborhoods mayor" was also a "walkable cities" enthusiast, so it's not surprising that around this same time, grassroots groups like Bike/Walk Nashville also appeared on the scene. To outsiders, though, their mission surely seemed unlikely. Music City's growth over the previous generation had sprawled across miles of Tennessee hillsides thanks to, and in celebration of, the Sunbelt's automobile culture.

The desire to buck those cultural tides—by Mayor Purcell, some of his aides, and a handful of local activists—may well have been why Nashville was awarded an Active Living By Design grant in 2003. Although local officials acknowledge that the $250,000 the city received through that project was not large, the money inspired them to think creatively about new ways to promote outdoor activity in Nashville.

Today, with those dollars long since spent, the spirit of the pilot project lives on in once-unlikely places. One such legacy is a green space along Mill Creek, at the edge of a populated neighborhood about five miles south of downtown's skyscrapers. After deadly floods raced through the Nashville area in 2010, a five-acre tract where several homes had been washed away and two others were badly damaged was bought by the city and reinvented as its first urban farm. Run by a nonprofit called Hands On Nashville, the farm on its far edge features wild growth and an absorbent wood-chip-and-gravel parking lot to mitigate future floods, but the rest is a patchwork quilt of vegetable beds and young fruit trees tended by hundreds of area school kids, in weekly visits or in a summer camp.

"We are always at the mercy of the elements," says Josh Corlew, the farm's program manager, sloshing through deep puddles as a torrential rain pounds his umbrella. He proudly shows off blueberry bushes, lettuce, and spinach growing through the winter in a long white tube; next are the wooden beds where flowers grow to attract beneficial insects to the farm, and where no chemicals are used. Corlew says that Hands On Nashville, aided by the city and some corporate donors, aims to teach young people to respect nutritional food, while offering its annual harvest to community groups that feed Nashville's poor. "When kids see where food comes from," Corlew says, "and they see it comes from the ground, the earth—then hopefully that will translate to greater respect for the environment."

Nashville's enthusiastic support for youth-oriented built environment projects like the urban farm came about through a combination of factors, including strong leadership from mayors like Purcell and the current incumbent, Karl Dean, who understand the importance of cohesive neighborhoods and an active lifestyle. Added to that is the dedication of a generation of planners who worked on those early projects and who have now moved into key decision-making jobs. For example, the newly minted college graduate who arrived in Nashville in the early 2000s as an enthusiastic urban planner to advance biking and walking—Adetokunbo "Toks" Omishakin—is now the chief of environment and planning for the Tennessee Department of Transportation, where he advocates for pedestrians and cyclists more broadly at the state level.

Omishakin says that in his early days as a Nashville planner promoting small neighborhood improvements such as bike lanes or crosswalks, his biggest roadblock was often engineers in the city's public works department who saw their job as moving as many cars as quickly as possible. Today the opposite is true. "I know they're champing at the bit to make these projects work," says Omishakin, adding that encouragement from residents pleading for amenities like new sidewalks has inspired a change in attitude. "All public servants want a pat on the back," he says. This reversal in the corridors of government explains why officials voice optimism about this second act, which includes a youth program called the Oasis Center.

On a dark December weeknight, with a frigid, soaking rain pummeling the outskirts of downtown Nashville, the search for this new generation of active living programs leads to Charlotte Avenue, a wide Sunbelt boulevard dotted with fast-food restaurants and a new barbecue joint. The Music City Bikeway—a twenty-six-mile bicycle route that runs up the avenue on its way toward the Tennessee State Capitol and the Cumberland

River—is understandably barren in the dark and the cold, but deep inside the bowels of a former khaki pants factory a half-dozen or so young cycling enthusiasts have found a shelter from the storm.

One of them is Max Cain, a wiry eighteen-year-old with a grey winter cap on his head and a shiny silver wrench in his hand. Organizers say he never misses the weekly workshop that is run by the Oasis Center, a multipurpose organization founded in 1969 to provide community-based care for young people experiencing alcohol and drug problems. Over the past four decades, it has evolved into one of the nation's leading youth-serving organizations, and offers twenty-one programs ranging from Nashville's only teen crisis shelter to Nashville's only college counseling center for first-generation college students. One of its programs, building on the momentum started by Active Living By Design during the 2000s, is its Bike Workshop. The workshop is open to any cycling enthusiast who wants to fix up a donated bike, with help from the long rows of hanging tools in this basement enclave and some friendly advice from the program director, Dan Furbish.

"I wanted to work with my hands," says Max Cain. "I wanted to work on bikes." Cain took the six-week bike-building and road-training course that Furbish has run for hundreds of mostly disadvantaged Nashville youth since 2009; then he just kept showing up when the course ended. Cain says he has rebuilt so many bikes he's lost count—maybe twenty, maybe forty—and his dad is yelling at him to get rid of the five or six that are cluttering their garage. Interning with Furbish, Cain is making plans to study auto repair. Meanwhile, he tours the city by bike. "I bicycle everywhere I go," he says, "except sometimes to school."

Local officials say that because the Oasis Center program targets kids in the Nashville school system, many of them from low-income minority families, it is emblematic of the growing push to encourage more diverse access to the bike trails and other projects launched in the 2000s. The program's organizers say that the built environment progress since Nashville received the

Foundation grant in 2003 has been nothing short of remarkable. Adams Carroll, who grew up in the Tennessee capital but developed his enthusiasm for bicycling in Oregon and Russia before returning to run the nonprofit Bike/Walk Nashville, says the first time he ever saw a dedicated bike lane in his hometown was in 2003. Public health experts say the region's car culture is a significant factor in Tennessee's having one of the highest obesity rates in United States.

As the focus has shifted toward fighting obesity, city and county health officials have taken on a bigger role in running local programs, often forging working alliances with transportation planners and public works engineers in ways that would have been unlikely a generation ago. An interesting example of the new paradigm is the work of planner Leslie Meehan at the region's Metropolitan Planning Organization, which sets priorities for spending federal dollars for transportation and related projects. There, Meehan created a position for herself that had not existed before: Director of Healthy Communities. "My focus is to look at the intersection of health and the built environment," she says. "That's pretty unique for a transportation agency."

Meehan's background is in health and wellness; she became interested in active living as a volunteer in a walk-to-school program in the late 1990s, and then worked as a City of Nashville planner on bike and pedestrian projects with Toks Omishakin in the mid-2000s. At the Metropolitan Planning Organization, Meehan says she has successfully sold her bosses on the notion that traffic and public health are closely linked. "We're able to take a more holistic approach so it works for transportation agencies," she says, "because we are required by federal law to address traffic fatalities and air pollution." But obesity is also increasingly on the minds of officials in Tennessee, she says.

Meehan has recently been involved in a thorny new issue that planners are taking up: school siting. Across much of the nation, but especially in the Sunbelt, communities increasingly locate schools on large, available, open tracts with plenty of room for cars; the downside is that these places are difficult for kids to walk to easily. (Further complicating matters: complex desegregation plans from the latter twentieth century that often involve long-distance busing.) Meehan says that poor school siting is another equity issue that falls heaviest on the poor and minorities: "If Mom and Dad don't have a car and you have to rely on the bus, then you can't easily participate in sports or cheerleading," she says. "But if you could walk, it would be a different story."

### Louisville, Kentucky

The path to active living is not always so smooth. In some communities, pilot programs funded through Active Living By Design have run into suspicion or distrust from politicians, residents, or local law enforcement, or into local issues such as crime or lack of funding for upkeep, problems that typically keep local residents indoors.

In 2006, the Robert Wood Johnson Foundation hired Lawrence D. Brown, a professor of health policy and management at Columbia University's Mailman School of Public Health, to evaluate four of the twenty-five Active Living By Design projects. According to Brown's report, one Foundation-funded project that seemed to epitomize the unanticipated early obstacles was the ACTIVE Louisville program run out of the city's housing authority to bring active living to a 725-unit Hope VI low-income housing project. (Hope VI is a plan developed by the US Department of Housing and Urban Development with the aim of revitalizing housing projects into mixed income developments. Its philosophy is based largely on the New Urbanism.)

In Kentucky's largest city, Brown discovered that legitimate fear of crime, and decades of distrust between neighborhoods, often thwarted the goal of fostering a walkable lifestyle for the city's poor, many of whom do not own cars. For example, greenways connecting the Hope VI development to other parts of Louisville were opposed, says one activist, by "older residents who fear rapists on trails and hooligans on bikes." Police officers who were asked to check on walking paths at night did not want to get out of their patrol cars. Planted trees were perceived as places where unsavory characters could hide. "The old idea that if you close off streets in public housing you'll deter drug dealing is wrong," one law-enforcement official told Brown. "Absence of traffic encourages drug dealing because we can't get so easily to where they congregate. And some dealers go around on bikes! To get at the dealers, you should trim back the trees, remove the shady spots, and so forth. The biggest active living challenge is getting people out."

In an interview following his study, Brown said there was a huge difference between what Louisville's health department or the middle-class planners wanted, and what the people who lived in the community wanted. He also found that entrenched business interests or car-culture traditionalists took advantage of multiple choke points in the political and planning processes, stopping or at least slowing down changes to the city's built environment. At the same time, however, Brown said that even in Louisville, where planners may have been overly optimistic in targeting such a disadvantaged community as their first big project, a growing population of outdoor enthusiasts started lobbying to add bike lanes or other amenities where conditions were more favorable.

"We really had a big goal and a tight timeline," says Nina Walfoort, who was program director of ACTIVE Louisville and is currently director of marketing and communications for the region's YMCA. She says there wasn't much time to prepare community groups for a concept that was new to many of them. But she also agrees with Brown's conclusion that ACTIVE Louisville did prepare the city for a current surge in built environment programs, under the leadership of a new health-oriented mayor who established a successor program in the city health department.

Today Louisville has an active walk-to-school program for kids and a number of built environment features such as pocket parks and wide streetscapes in a newer downtown redevelopment project. It has negotiated a shared-use agreement for the sports facilities at an east side high school. "A lot of seeds were planted," Walfoort says. "It caused a lot of cross-pollination and partnerships."

## —⁓— Other Communities

In other communities studied by Columbia's Lawrence Brown, the common obstacles tended to be politicians, developers (who were also the politicians' donors), and bureaucrats who'd succeeded under the traditional rules of real estate and sometimes had a rocky relationship with unconventional Smart Growth advocates. But each Active Living program also faced uniquely local barriers.

In the economically struggling Rust Belt community of Wilkes-Barre, Pennsylvania, the local Chamber of Commerce viewed the conversion of abandoned coal rail lines to outdoor walking and biking trails as a cornerstone of economic redevelopment. But the project suffered, because in that cash-poor community, grants to build new trails did not come with money to maintain them against such strains as northeast Pennsylvania's rugged weather. And in Albuquerque, one planner described most post-1990 development to Brown as "walled-in subdivisions like feudal villages." Against that mindset, such tame proposals as a few "Great Streets" to accommodate pedestrians and cyclists, with wide sidewalks fronting unique stores and restaurants with outdoor tables, drew skepticism—even hostility. Said one resident of the "Great Streets" concept: "That's fine for my twenty-year-old daughter, but I'm not leaving my car at home."

Still, as the first decade of built environment projects wound down, dozens of cities across the country—especially those with energetic, pro-activity mayors and civic leadership—looked past some of the early obstacles and sought to adopt and expand on best practices, some of which were developed in Active Living By Design demonstration cities such as Buffalo and Nashville.

One of the new advocates is Chip Johnson, the mayor of Hernando, Mississippi, a small but fast-growing exurban community about twenty-five miles south of Memphis. The former owner of a carpet-cleaning business, Johnson had little background in public health when he became mayor in 2005, but his perspective radically changed after he attended a Southern Obesity Summit, partially funded by the Foundation, that laid out some of the successful strategies for combating obesity. Returning home, Johnson tackled the issue with the zeal of a convert. Although Hernando did not even have a parks department when he became mayor, Johnson successfully pushed for programs that might improve health in the community. These included a weekly farmers' market, a community garden, enacting a Complete Streets ordinance, and building a mile of new sidewalk that connects a low-income neighborhood to an elementary school.

In an interview, Johnson said he was proud that, in fiscally conservative Mississippi, some of his more effective measures have cost very little. "State law requires that motorists give bicyclists a three-foot berth," he says, "so we have posted that on signs all over the town . . . so people understand that cyclists have a right. We're changing a lot of the mindset." Today, Johnson and Hernando use the town's newfound reputation—it was the first community to be cited as the state's "Healthiest Hometown" by the Blue Cross & Blue Shield of Mississippi Foundation—as an economic development tool. Johnson says an employer from a neighboring county just relocated a hundred employees to Hernando, and not because of tax incentives; the employer simply saw Hernando as a good place for workers to live and raise their families.

Not surprisingly, some of the hot spots of built environment progressivism are cities like Seattle and Portland, Oregon, places that have received an influx of highly educated young urban enthusiasts who don't need to be sold on the benefits of an active lifestyle. And in New York City, under recently departed mayor Michael Bloomberg, the city launched the privately backed Citi Bike program that has put nearly six thousand shareable bicycles in 330 locations, while pushing for changes in the building code that would require open stairways with signs to encourage people to walk.

But, says Active Living Research's Sallis, dynamic mayors have also put the built environment on the map in such car-dominated Sunbelt municipalities as Oklahoma City. There, popular Mayor Mick Cornett—jolted into action by a 2007 magazine article stating that his city had one of nation's highest obesity rates—led Oklahoma City to float bonds and pass a sales tax increase that together have financed more than three hundred miles of sidewalks, more than thirty-two miles of bike trails, a riverfront park, and other outdoor amenities.

Even so, as a late 2013 article in Cornett's hometown *Oklahoma Gazette* reported, obesity remains disturbingly high in Oklahoma City. It affects one in three adults, ranking the city sixth worst in the nation among large cities, according to the CDC.

This begs a question raised by some public-health researchers as childhood obesity became a focus of the built environment movement: if weight loss is now the primary purpose of building bike trails or encouraging children to walk to school, how will scientists produce evidence-based findings of what works best, when exercise is just one among several factors, along with diet and heredity, that can determine an individual's body mass?

Sallis concedes the difficulty in making one-to-one correlations between finished built environment projects and weight loss in a community. But he notes that the swift rise of childhood obesity rates in the latter twentieth century and the 2000s all but mandated trying a variety of approaches on a large scale, rather than waiting on small-batch academic research. "There's concern that this is a long-term problem," says Sallis, "and if you attack just one area, that might not be sufficient." He and other researchers have been encouraged by data that started to emerge by 2012 showing a drop in childhood obesity rates in several large cities with aggressive active living and healthy eating programs.

Philadelphia, a pioneer in locating new supermarkets in low-income neighborhoods, saw obesity among school children decline by 5 percent between 2006 and 2010, according to the city's Department of Public Health, which found a steeper drop among black than white children. In other areas, including Mississippi, child obesity rates also fell during the same period, but the rates fell faster for white kids than for black kids. That has provoked an even greater sense of urgency to advocates seeking more equity in healthy eating and lifestyle programs.

## —∿— Conclusion

Over the last five years, the enthusiasm among a growing number of urban leaders and their constituents for bike lanes or walkable neighborhoods has met countervailing forces—the governmental budget crunch that hit after the 2008 fiscal crisis, as well as an alliance between conservative antispending factions—typified by, but not limited to, the Tea Party movement—and politicians on the right side of the spectrum. With some critics branding built environment projects as costly and unnecessary "social engineering," supporters of active living efforts have become more creative in winning political support and the dollars that come with it.

Part of the problem, experts agree, is that fiscal conservatism is strongest in Sunbelt states where obesity rates are the highest. Advocates like Hernando mayor Johnson—who has used parks and green space to attract new employers to his Mississippi community—say that the best and sometimes the only way to sell the built environment agenda to wary politicians is by promoting its value in creating jobs. Built environment projects are not just public works projects, he says; they are also infrastructure improvements that make a community more attractive to residents or business owners.

"Their perspective is, 'Is this a job creator?'" says Phil Bors, the senior project officer for Active Living By Design in Chapel Hill. Jobs are often seen as more important to communities than improving health. Hampden County, Massachusetts, for example, responded to its less than stellar place in the County Health Rankings by focusing all of its attention on one thing: jobs. Longtime built environment advocates take pride that a privately owned Web site called Walk Score now rates homes on the market for their ease in walking to school or shopping, and this rating is increasingly touted in real estate ads.

At the same time, there is widespread agreement that gains in walkability have so far reached more affluent neighborhoods than communities struggling with poverty. Sarah Strunk, who serves as the national program director of both Active Living By Design and Healthy Kids, Healthy Communities, says she's very much aware of where more work is required. She singles out the problem of equity—that is, bringing physical improvements to poorer neighborhoods where political power is low and problems such as crime persist. Another problem is that the United States remains very much a car culture.

But despite these and other challenges, much has been learned from the built environment programs, and the importance of the physical environment is more widely recognized than before. Local, state, and federal governments are now spending millions of dollars to follow up on the promise and lessons learned from early built environment pilot projects. Young people are driving less than they had previously—preferring to take public transportation, walk, or bike. And it has become easier to tackle problems like tight budgets, pro-automobile bias, or the equity gap because a dozen years of built environment experimentation have resulted in a new generation of enlightened community planners and health officials, as well as engaged citizens.

One of those people is Ian Thomas, who in the late 1990s moved to the university town of Columbia, Missouri. So dismayed was he at how difficult it was to get around on a bicycle that he founded a group called PedNet, which received an Active Living By Design grant. Thomas and others were then able to parlay the Foundation's initial $200,000 investment into a $25 million federal demonstration grant to build bike trails. Today, Thomas, who surrendered his role as executive director of PedNet to run for public office as "an experienced community builder," represents the Fourth Ward on the Columbia City Council.

# The Healthy Schools Program

*Paul Jablow*

## Introduction

Throughout much of its first four decades, the Robert Wood Johnson Foundation chose to fund health clinics in primary and secondary schools. In 1978, the Foundation funded the School Health Services Program, which used nurse practitioners to provide services, with physicians providing backup. Since that time, the Foundation has invested more than $64 million in school health clinics.

In an interview for the Foundation's oral history, Catherine DeAngelis, who was director of the School Health Services Program and later the editor in chief of the *Journal of the American Medical Association*, said, "The whole issue of school health, in one way, is a very old concept in pediatrics. At the turn of the [nineteenth] century, taking care of the immigrant kids in New York happened in the schools."

Not only is this an old concept, but it also reflects a narrow view of the role of schools in children's health: the school clinic as an extension of the health care system. More recent thought regards schools as places to improve the health of children, as schools are where children spend most of their time, and where they have meals and get exercise.

This is the view that the Foundation has taken. It has invested $32 million in Playworks, a program using AmeriCorps volunteers to organize recess time in schools in low-income neighborhoods.[1] It invested even more— $51 million—in the Healthy Schools Program, carried out in conjunction with the Clinton Foundation and the American Heart Association. As Paul Jablow reports, the Healthy Schools Program has already helped more than twenty-four thousand schools bring more nutritious food and greater opportunities for physical activity to their school children.

Paul Jablow is a freelance writer who spent thirty years as a reporter and editor for *The Philadelphia Inquirer*. In addition to writing for the *Anthology*, he is the author of several of the Foundation's program results reports.

## Note

1. C. Newbergh, "Playworks/Sports4Kids," in S. L. Isaacs and D. C. Colby (eds.), *To Improve Health and Health Care: The Robert Wood Johnson Foundation Anthology*, Vol. XIV (San Francisco: Jossey-Bass, 2011).

The Oklahoma sky was gloomy, with a hint of rain in the autumn air, as the students at Roosevelt Elementary School in Pryor circled the patchy grass yard, some at a leisurely amble, others elbowing their way ahead at a faster pace. Some carried backpacks, some wore T-shirts or Halloween costumes despite the early morning chill, but they all stopped briefly in front of assistant principal David Miller to get one of the wooden Popsicle sticks he was handing out from a bag. Once back inside, the students would give the sticks to their classroom teachers for credit toward their goal of walking one hundred miles.

Later that morning, Miller observed Sara Melugin's class where the kids rocked back and forth at their desks on large, inflated "stability balls" that gave them small bits of exercise and helped them work off typical fourth-grade fidgetiness. Then, at lunch hour, the kindergarten students filed out of the lunchroom to witness a strange sight indeed—a bicycle attached to a blender as maintenance man Conrad Gunter pedaled furiously, mixing a healthy fruit shake.

Just two years before, the students would have started their day hanging out in the breakfast room instead of with a fitness walk. Melugin's class would have been seated at standard desks. And, of course, no one would have even *heard* of a "fender blender" bicycle.

School secretary Sheri Madole says that the morning exercise walks have already helped her grandson's ADHD symptoms. Melugin says her students "are focusing better" with the fitness balls. And kindergartener Johnny "Junior" Jeffries says that when he got home after school that day, he would ask his mother, "Will you make a slushie for me?"

These small victories for physical fitness and wellness took place at a rural school in Pryor, forty miles northeast of Tulsa. But for the Alliance for a Healthier Generation, the joint initiative of the American Heart Association and the Clinton Foundation that started the Healthy Schools Program in 2006—and for the Robert Wood Johnson Foundation, which has supported it with grants totaling roughly $51 million—the hope is that such lessons will be multiplied thousands of times over in schools across the country, all in the name of chipping away at the goal of reversing the epidemic of childhood obesity by 2015.

By mid-2014, more than twenty-four thousand schools, including Roosevelt, had participated in the program, which has reached more than twelve million students. Howell Wechsler, CEO of the Alliance for a Healthier Generation, says he thinks the program can reach its goal of thirty thousand schools by the end of 2015.

## —⌇— A Lesson Taken to Heart

As Wechsler tells it, it all started with Bill Clinton's diagnosis of heart disease. Stricken with an angina attack in September 2004, the former president underwent quadruple bypass surgery four days later and was told that he had probably been months away from what most likely would have been a fatal heart attack.

"He attributed his health problems at a relatively young age [fifty-eight] to mistakes he'd made in his diet," says Wechsler. The leadership of the American Heart Association contacted Clinton during his recuperation. They wondered how to use the former president's high visibility to focus attention on the issue and persuade Americans to take better care of themselves. "They didn't want to do some public relations event," Wechsler says, "but something that would have real impact."

The following year, the American Heart Association and the William J. Clinton Foundation formed the Alliance for a Healthier Generation, a campaign to change the lifestyles of America's children decades before they became candidates for the operating table. Or, as Clinton and others said at the time, before they became the first generation in US history to live shorter lives than their parents.

Trooper Sanders, then the domestic policy adviser for the Clinton Foundation, says that schools were targeted as an Alliance initiative for two reasons. First, it was a way to reach communities across the country, "to demonstrate change that could be scaled broadly." Second, the Clinton Foundation had a model, its fight against HIV/AIDs in Africa, to build on.

Since 2002, the Clinton Foundation had worked with the pharmaceutical industry, governments, and nongovernmental organizations to make medicines less expensive and more widely available. Now, the Alliance would be working with the food and beverage industries and school districts to make healthy foods more widely available.

So the Alliance opened negotiations with major players in the food industry and started looking for funding for the program. Ira Magaziner, who had advised Hillary Clinton on health reform in the early 1990s and who was head of the Clinton Foundation's global health initiatives, immediately thought of the Robert Wood Johnson Foundation. He had worked in the White House with Risa Lavizzo-Mourey, the Foundation's president and chief executive officer, back when she was a member of the President's Task Force on National Health Care Reform and a consultant on health policy. "I knew she had a passion about this," says Magaziner, "and I knew the Robert Wood Johnson Foundation was doing some leading work in this area. We were new in the field, but we knew we could make a difference."

Magaziner phoned Lavizzo-Mourey and suggested a partnership around the Healthy Schools Program. The idea went hand in hand with her goal to reverse childhood obesity. "Childhood obesity was an issue people had been watching from the sidelines for a while," says Lavizzo-Mourey. "It was seen as an intractable problem because it required systems change on a daily basis." In contrast, she says, the Foundation's fight against smoking had been less complicated because "if you quit smoking, you quit smoking. Or you don't start. But you've got to eat."

As childhood obesity rates soared, the Foundation's staff increasingly saw schools as critical in the effort to reduce childhood obesity. "School is where the kids are," says Jim Marks, senior vice president of the Robert Wood Johnson Foundation. "It's where they spend their time and where they're often inactive." Children may take half their meals at schools, he explains, at least during the academic year, and those meals may comprise more than half of their daily caloric intake. "There are two ways you invest in people—health and education," he says. "And they're centrally linked, especially at the childhood level."

The Foundation awarded the Alliance a start-up grant of $8 million, and in May 2006 Ginny Ehrlich, a veteran public health and education professional, was named CEO of the Healthy Schools Program. Ehrlich had previously founded Oregon's Healthy Kids Learn Better Partnership, a public-private coalition comprising five state agencies, state and local education policymakers, and more than forty nongovernmental organizations. She welcomed the challenge, in part because childhood obesity is not a problem that occurs in isolation: "If you look at the kids who are disproportionately affected by the obesity epidemic," says Ehrlich, "they are kids who are living in poverty." They are also, she says, kids who are less likely to be from intact homes. Or whose parents are working at low-wage jobs.

The components of the first Robert Wood Johnson Foundation grant included:

- Physical activity and nutrition standards for schools
- A technical assistance program to help schools meet those standards
- A staff wellness program
- A recognition program for schools that made healthy changes

Ehrlich saw staff wellness as a key component. "We wanted to see the adults who were role models in those kids' lives walking the talk, so to speak." She also wanted the program to draw on the most advanced research while still being understandable to classroom teachers. "They don't deal with the world of journals and academia," Ehrlich says. "You have to give them reason to believe."

## —∿— Getting Started

The American Heart Association had already recruited almost two hundred schools to participate in the new project. Ehrlich and her staff added another thirty-one as they drew up the design for the program. Then they appointed an advisory group consisting of about twenty school officials, educational experts, specialists in physical education and nutrition, and staff members of the Centers for Disease Control and Prevention. Then staff from the Alliance, the American Heart Association, and the Foundation began drawing up recommended nutrition guidelines for the schools.

By 2006, the Alliance had developed guidelines for competitive foods and beverages—those offered in addition to regular school meals. They specified, for example, that beverages for elementary school children be limited to bottled water, eight-ounce servings of 100 percent juice, and eight-ounce servings of fat-free or low-fat milk. The Alliance and the American Beverage Association signed an agreement stipulating that the beverage association would "limit the number of calories available in beverages" and give students "even more low-calorie, nutritious, smaller-portion choices." According to one assessment, between 2004 and the 2009–2010 school year, the beverage industry had reduced the caloric content of the soft drinks shipped to schools by 90 percent.[1]

The agreement with the American Beverage Association was the first in a series of agreements that the Alliance would sign with the food industry, culminating in the 2011 agreement with fourteen food manufacturers, technology companies, and group purchasing organizations to provide more healthy options for school meals.

In 2010, First Lady Michelle Obama announced her "Let's Move!" initiative, throwing the prestige of her position behind improving the quality of food in schools, making healthy foods more affordable and accessible for families, and focusing more on physical education. After the federal Healthy, Hunger-Free Kids Act of 2010 became law, Ehrlich says the Alliance worked closely with the US Department of Agriculture (USDA) as it was formulating its guidelines.

The initial Foundation grant for the Healthy Schools Program did not specify the number of schools to be reached. By May 2007, the program was providing hands-on technical assistance to 230 schools and online support to 900 more. In August 2007, the Foundation raised the stakes with a $20 million grant to expand the program to at least 6,400 schools. Then, in the fall of 2011—with more than 10,000 schools now enrolled—the Foundation awarded the Alliance another $23 million to continue the program through the end of November 2014.

## —∿— How the Healthy Schools Program Works

The Healthy Schools Program provides online and on-site technical support to schools across the country in what program leaders describe as the schools' "efforts to engage the entire school community—including administrators, parents, and school vendors." A quarter of the schools receive on-site technical assistance, while three-quarters receive online technical support.

The work is based on the Healthy Schools Program Framework, a set of best-practice guidelines developed with the help of the program's national panel of experts. The guidelines, which serve as a roadmap for creating a healthier school environment, form the basis of the National Recognition Award, which is presented to schools at the bronze, silver, and gold levels based on policy and program changes made in seven separate areas:

- Policy/Systems
- Employee Wellness

- School Meals
- Physical Education
- Competitive Foods and Beverages
- Student Wellness
- Health Education

To reach the bronze level in school meals, for example, a school must serve both breakfast and lunch, with food meeting USDA standards for reimbursable meals and a different vegetable served every day. In addition, there has to have been annual staff training for all food service personnel.

For the silver level, additional requirements include serving non-fried fish at least once a week and serving either no desserts or only desserts meeting Alliance Competitive Foods Guidelines.

For the gold level, the bar is raised to require schools to offer "only lean protein products such as lean red meat, skinless poultry, fat-free, lean deli meats, fat-free or low-fat cheese, beans, tofu, etc."

Schools that reach any of the award levels are invited by the Alliance to send representatives to their annual recognition ceremony, usually at the Clinton Library in Little Rock, Arkansas, with the former president speaking. But while winning a bronze, silver, or gold is nice, the real goal for these schools is long-term sustainable change.

Schools in the program are urged to follow a six-step regimen that starts with forming a school wellness council that includes students, faculty, and representatives from the community, and then taking a Healthy Schools Program inventory of their current wellness efforts. The program works through school districts, says Brian Weaver, the Healthy Schools Program vice president, because buy-in from the district level as well as the school level is seen as vital.

Schools receive on-site technical assistance with program staff members called "relationship managers." They start with three "train the trainer" introductory sessions in the fall of the first year, after which the relationship managers connect the schools with other resources, such as experts in the health and wellness field; hold workshops and webinars; speak at district or regional events; and perhaps help them with an awards application.

Amanda Green, a regional director for eight states in the Midwest, estimates that every school has contact with the program at least once a month during the school year. All schools also have access to a panel of six nationally recognized experts on physical activity, nutrition, wellness, and policy changes.

"We have to be seen as a resource that's not going away," says Brian Weaver. Schools are expected to "graduate" out of the on-site program in four years, and at that point, the hope is that "we've left them with an infrastructure so they can continue to address health and wellness issues."

## —∾— The Healthy Schools Program in Practice

As the case studies below indicate, although they all operated within the Healthy Schools Program's guidelines, no two schools or school districts took exactly the same approach.

### Pryor, Oklahoma

For three decades, Laura Holloway had coached basketball, track, and softball at high schools and junior high schools in Texas and in her native Oklahoma. Her track athletes had won some thirty state championships. Then, during the 2010–2011 school year, Holloway met John Ratey and realized that coaching in and of itself would never again be enough for her.

It was at a meeting of the national association for physical education teachers in San Diego that Holloway heard a talk by Ratey, a clinical psychiatrist at Harvard Medical School. He told the assembled physical education teachers how vital exercise was for the brain; he also discussed the damage that a sedentary lifestyle was doing not just to people's bodies, but also to their brains.

At around the same time, Holloway had heard the saying that today's students were part of the first generation of Americans who would be less healthy than their parents. Between that statement and Ratey's talk, something clicked in her. "Sometimes you just hear statements that hit you," she says. "Up until that time, I had always been around the athletic side of things.... This generation is different. We have so much non-movement because of technology."

When she returned to Oklahoma, Holloway told district superintendent Don Raleigh that she wanted to shift her focus to the entire student population. And she wanted to do it in Pryor, where she was born and raised. Raleigh, still new in the superintendent's job, is a great admirer of Stephen R. Covey's best-selling 1989 book *The 7 Habits of Highly Effective People,* and particularly of the seventh habit, "Sharpen the Saw." For Covey, that meant, "Balance and renew your resources, energy, and health to create a sustainable, long-term, effective lifestyle."

It was not surprising, then, that Holloway found Raleigh an easy sell. "We're in a state that hasn't had a lot of success on wellness indexes," Raleigh says. "I don't think health and fitness has been a priority of too many families here." He began gathering resources and local support to change the district's culture and spread that change into the community. "We wanted kids to take responsibility for their choices," he says.

Raleigh won community support for bond issues to build gymnasiums at two elementary schools. And he named Holloway director of health and wellness for the five-school, 2,700-student district and gave her the go-ahead to work for change throughout the system. "You don't pull back a racehorse," says Raleigh.

In 2010, Holloway wrote a proposal for a Carol M. White Physical Education Program grant from the US Department of Education. It was rejected. The following year she succeeded. She then brought the district into the Healthy Schools Program. The district next instituted "Walking Wednesdays," in which parents drive their kids to designated church or local business parking lots about a half-mile from school and walk the rest of the way together. The district also initiated a Weight Watchers program for the staff.

"Wellness isn't just one more thing to add on," Raleigh says, "and I think our teachers are learning that." The district converted an empty room in the junior high school into a fitness center and trained all teachers to incorporate wellness into their classrooms. This included regular "brain breaks"—for example, stopping classes for a few minutes so everyone can exercise to videos. The district instituted the SPARK fitness curriculum, bought hands-on exercise equipment, such as Hula Hoops, for all students, and built climbing walls in the elementary schools and junior high schools. The schools have also worked with the Cherokee Nation's Wings running program—the district's student population is 44 percent Native American.

In the near future, says Holloway, the district hopes to add an activity-based movement lab in the high school for students to use before testing—hopefully to improve performance—or to reduce stress after testing. "It's kind of like a decompressor for them," she says. Beyond that, the district's goal is more ambitious: "We want wellness to be such an ingrained part of our culture," says district superintendent Raleigh, "that we don't know we're doing it."

### Elizabeth, New Jersey

There's a poster outside the principal's office at Terence C. Reilly Elementary School No. 7 in Elizabeth, New Jersey, with the dates of staff birthdays and pictures of cupcakes. Just don't try getting a real one through the school entrance. Not on Jennifer Cedeño's watch.

Since her appointment as principal at the end of 2008, Cedeño has taken this school in a gritty, inner-city neighborhood from a place of cheesecake fundraisers and recesses that just broke up the school day to one of six winners of the Healthy Schools Program gold-level award.

"The culture of the district was not one of health and wellness," says Cedeño. But now all schools in the district are in the program; and at Reilly, wellness is threaded through the classrooms, the gym, and the cafeteria like the pattern of an intricate tapestry. The change doesn't stop there. If the lessons from the school don't make it outside to the students' homes, Cedeño says, she hasn't done her job: "The future is doing health care and wellness with families."

Inside the school, the change is visible in the classrooms, in the halls, and during recess. In a fourth-grade health class, PE and health education teacher Beatriz Villarino-Kong has the kids determine the number of calories in a bag of Oreos by multiplying the number of servings by the number of calories in each, adding a brief lesson on how to read a food label. Belinda Jimenez divides the kids in her seventh-grade health class into four groups for a smoothie-blending contest in which they try to mask the flavor of a vegetable with other ingredients, including yogurt and fresh fruit. "I actually know how many calories I'm mixing," says Heidy Tejeda, age twelve. She says she has taken some of the healthy cooking lessons home to her family. "Do they like it?" she is asked. "They appreciate it," she says, after a tactful pause.

A blare of music echoes throughout the school and students spill out into the hallways, doing jumping jacks in the daily "Jam-a-Minute" exercise break. Cedeño, a tall, slender woman who grew up in Queens, New York, and has spent the last fifteen years in Elizabeth, eagerly joins in, heels clicking on the freshly lacquered floor.

Recess is a blur of noisy activity, students running and jumping from exercise station to exercise station. Physical education teacher Jairo Labrador sees a student using incorrect form doing sit-ups on an exercise ball and walks over to correct her. Labrador says he teaches students in an elective exercise science class how to design their own exercise circuits using readily available materials.

Elizabeth is not a wealthy district, and with 85 percent of Reilly's students eligible for free or reduced-price lunches, there is hardly a financial surplus for Cedeño to tap into. But she scrounged for other funds, getting grants to turn what had been a storage room into a gleaming dance studio. And like many principals in challenging economic environments, she looks for versatility on her staff. Sixth-grade social studies teacher Michelle Pedrayes, for example, also teaches ballet.

Cedeño also looks for ways to take the school's health culture out into the community, with offerings including Zumba nights and cooking classes in which parents in the heavily Hispanic district are given healthier recipes for tacos and other dishes. While Elizabeth has several supermarkets, Cedeño says that the parents often avoid them in favor of bodegas; she encourages them to look for healthy food choices wherever they can find them. "Some of the students say their parents are cooking better," Cedeño says. "I see it in what comes here in lunchboxes, or at birthday parties."

Davida Gurstelle, the Alliance's regional director for the greater New York City area, holds workshops on healthy fundraisers—no sweets involved—attended by several schools "so the district won't have to reinvent the wheel." Some of the results can be seen at a meeting of the Reilly Elementary School wellness council. After faculty, student, and community members cover an agenda including a breast cancer awareness run, a wellness fair, and planning for National Nutrition Month activities, several of the student members, all thirteen-year-old eighth graders, explain why wellness isn't just a personal matter to them. Jasmine Ruckert says she's concerned about numerous health issues in her family; to help them change, she's started giving cooking lessons at home. Gabriel Trigo, who is of Portuguese descent, says that at his urging, his family is now following their ancestral Mediterranean diet. "We've gone back to our roots," he says. "Eating healthy."

For many of the students, says Cedeño, this is not an easy option. When Friday arrives and school meals have ended, some of the lowest-income students must bring home canned goods from food pantries, and those often aren't healthy choices. "It's better than nothing," she says, "but it's not the best."

The best is what Jennifer Cedeño is always looking for. "I feel we do the job in here," she says. "The future is outside the walls."

### Queens, New York

Almost invariably, new entrants in the Healthy Schools Program face major changes in introducing and then adjusting to a culture of wellness. But what if someone started a school from scratch built around that theme?

As a kindergarten teacher in a Harlem charter school, Robert Groff was pondering just that a few years ago as he did a research project on healthy lifestyles for his certification as a school principal. "It just made sense," Groff recalls thinking. And in 2008, it became a reality—a four-story, two-toned brick building in a bustling, predominantly Chinese community in Flushing, Queens.

The Active Learning Elementary School (TALES) is in a low-income area, with some two-thirds of its students eligible for free or reduced-price lunches. Most of the kids come in speaking only Mandarin, but when they leave they are fluent in both English and wellness. "They have the ability to talk about it," says Groff, the school's principal. "If they're in third grade, it's been part of their life since Pre-K." In 2013, TALES became the first New York City school to offer an all-vegetarian lunch menu, a cross-cultural medley featuring such items as vegetarian chili with brown rice, falafel, roasted tofu with Asian sesame sauce, sweet potato fries, and plantains.

One parent, Karen Lee, says the dietary change at TALES has had major benefits for her daughter Caitlin, who is in first grade. A very picky eater, Caitlin had chronic constipation and low muscle tone for years, and nutritionists consulted by the family urged a more varied diet.

But Caitlin became willing only after she saw her classmates at TALES trying new foods. "It was a gradual process," says Lee. "They talked about food in class and my daughter said, 'I want to try a carrot,' or 'I want to try a tomato.' Her symptoms improved in six months." She was also stronger on the playground, no longer having to stop at the first rung of the monkey bars—now she can handle all six rungs.

The program has had an added benefit. At a family night at the school, parents, grandparents, and caregivers joined the children and shared the vegetarian menu. Lee's husband, "the biggest red meat eater" prior to that evening, liked the food so much that he went back for seconds. And TALES second grade teacher Jacqueline Mark, who previously taught in the South Bronx, says she sees the difference in the kids' classroom alertness. "I'm familiar with bug juice and Doritos for breakfast," she says. "The kids here are definitely more focused. They know what they're doing and why."

A silver level school, TALES has shown significant improvements in body mass index, or BMI. From fall 2011 to spring 2012, two-thirds of the overweight or obese children improved, and the number of obese or underweight children was reduced by 4.5 percent. Robert Groff cites the school's partnerships with such groups as FAN4Kids, which provides on-site physical education and nutrition instruction, and the New York Coalition for Healthy School Food. Also, Geri Wurman, who heads the Healthy Schools Program in New York and Connecticut, helped connect the school with local resources to further their interest in community gardening; she held professional development sessions that TALES staff attended twice a year; and she obtained free books on healthy eating for parents attending family nights.

At TALES, there has been no shortage of sweat equity involved: Groff personally built a sandbox in the schoolyard and planted apple and pear trees. He is also seeking funds for a research project on TALES graduates to see whether BMI improvements from the school years are sustained over time. In the future, says Groff, "We want to help someone else start this in another place."

## Kearney, Nebraska

The Kearney, Nebraska, district is one that the Alliance and the Robert Wood Johnson Foundation point to as a success story. Obesity rates declined 22 percent in grades K–5 between 2006 and 2013. Carol S. Renner, associate superintendent of Kearney Public Schools, calls the decline the result of a "village effort" that included improving local parks by creating a new playground, building new splash parks, revitalizing swimming pools, and developing a partnership between a local hospital and a physicians' group to support student fitness activities.

Considerable progress had already been made by the time the district joined the Healthy Schools Program in 2008. In 2006, for example, the district had started working with Kate Heelan, a professor of exercise science at the University of Nebraska at Kearney and a mother of children in the district, to track student BMI. Most districts do not do this, says Healthy Schools vice president Brian Weaver, for reasons of both privacy and a lack of trained personnel.

In 2008, the district was awarded a $900,000 Carol M. White Physical Education Program grant to improve the schools' physical education programs. So when Healthy Schools Program regional manager Shannon Vogler began working with the schools, their attack on the obesity epidemic was well under way, and she saw her goal as taking them to the next level. "Many schools do a lot of nice things," says Vogler, "but they don't have a roadmap. We offered a clear framework of best practices and training."

The Physical Education Program grant dealt only with physical education, so when the Healthy Schools Program got under way, Vogler started working with the district's staff on all aspects of its framework. She guided the schools through a competitive process to get free training and discounted physical education curriculum materials, and she helped them raise funds. In addition, she worked with the schools to incorporate physical activity breaks into the classroom. The Healthy Schools Program instituted nights for parents to learn healthy recipes and cooking techniques, and collaborated with the University on developing and implementing a health education curriculum.

In the 2012–2013 school year, Central Elementary piloted a daily physical education class as opposed to one taking place only two or three days a week. "It was a huge success," says district school nurse Julene Lesher. "Besides a boost in learning power from extra physical activity, we immediately noticed a decrease in disruptive behaviors and a reduction in student visits to the health room. Daily PE also allowed extra collaboration and planning time for classroom teachers." Lesher developed a staff manual aimed at bringing new personnel up to speed on school wellness efforts. "The challenge is keeping wellness at the forefront," she says. "New staffers and new administrators bring in the health habits they had at other schools."

In 2011, four of the eleven Kearney schools participating in the Healthy Schools Program received bronze recognition. "What made this happen isn't unique," says Shannon Vogler. "There's no magic bullet."

## —ᗣᗧ— Conclusion

Any judgment on how effective the Healthy Schools Program has been will depend to some extent on how one measures effectiveness. If the goal has been to change the culture in participating schools, the answer is that the program has largely had a positive impact. Walk into a school like Roosevelt, Reilly, or TALES, and you know you're in a very different universe from that of conventional public schools. The energy is different, the wall charts and slogans are different, and many of the student, teacher, and staff activities are different. "When I teach an hour-long class, I start to lose them twenty-five to thirty minutes into it," says Julene Lesher, the Kearney school nurse. "I have them do a one-minute activity break, and after that they are alert and engaged once again."

But deeper questions remain. Does it make the kids healthier? Will it give them the tools to remain healthier as they move into the adult world? Will more schools buy into it? Research into the effects of school-based interventions on wellness and BMI is described by those working in the field as "promising, but mixed." Schools are an important influence, but students are exposed to many other influences: home, their peers, advertising, and the fast-food culture, among others. "The schools cannot do it alone," says researcher Jamie Chriqui, a nationally recognized expert on childhood obesity. "If we don't focus on the broader environment, all the inroads we're making in schools will be lost. Schools are just one piece of the obesity environment."

In 2011, the RMC Research Corporation of Portland, Oregon, conducted an evaluation of the Healthy Schools Program. The evaluation included on-site visits to a random sampling of twenty-one schools starting in the program prior to the 2011–12 school year. Here are some of RMC's findings:

- Nearly 70 percent of the schools using the on-site model moved up at least one recognition level in at least one of the eight content areas. Thirty percent reached the overall award level.

- Evidence was "inconclusive" for schools using the online model.

- Significant declines in BMI were reported in middle schools but not in elementary or high schools.

- Schools with high proportions of African American or Hispanic students demonstrated significantly more progress in program implementation than other schools, as did schools located in the South.

The evaluation concluded that "The first five years of the Healthy Schools Program provide strong evidence that the program's technical assistance and training model is effective with schools participating in the onsite program."

Alliance CEO Howell Wechsler is not surprised that the most progress in reducing BMI came in middle schools, since middle-school students start out at a lower level than elementary school students. "Some of the practices may be better in elementary schools," he says. "They may be getting more physical education, and they have less access to junk foods. In middle school, it's a whole new world opening up to them. There's less regimented PE, more access to junk foods." As for high school students, they're "a tough nut to crack," says Wechsler. "By that age, patterns are set."

To obtain more precise answers to questions about what works and what doesn't, and from a larger group of people, in 2013 the Foundation commissioned Kristine Madsen, an assistant professor of public health at the University of California, Berkeley, to conduct a study of the Healthy Schools Program's impact on student BMI in California. California has collected BMI data on students in grades five, seven, and nine since 2005. Madsen's study will examine data going back to 2005 and will include students from schools in both the on-site and online Healthy Schools Programs, as well as students whose schools are involved in neither.

Meanwhile, questions have arisen as to whether or not BMI is even the proper indicator of the Healthy Schools Program's effectiveness. "The most important outcome to be examined for a program such as Healthy Schools is whether the school's policies and environment have been changed," Howell Wechsler says. "Any impact on outcomes such as dietary or physical activity behaviors, fitness or weight status, or academic measures should be explored, though not necessarily expected." While not all Healthy Schools Program participants are as successful as Roosevelt, Reilly, and TALES, most schools do stick with the on-site program once they're in it. Schools receiving online technical assistance drop out at a higher rate than those receiving on-site assistance.

The biggest obstacle of all, however, has been the reluctance of schools to even sign up, mainly because of the variety of pressures they face in the current educational environment. "Principals are scared to take even one minute away from testing," says the Healthy Schools Program's Geri Wurman. Lisa Perry, the Alliance's national physical education and physical activity adviser, notes, "We've seen a pretty dramatic decline in physical education over the years. If they've got to cut something, they cut art, music, and physical education."

The key to selling wellness programs to overburdened, cash-strapped principals and school districts is to show them the academic benefits, advises the childhood obesity researcher Jamie Chriqui. "Unless it helps them improve the academic bottom line," she says, "they're going to be resistant."

"When we started," says Robert Wood Johnson Foundation CEO Risa Lavizzo-Mourey, "folks said, 'You can't burden the schools with one more thing.' It was common wisdom. But from where I sit, the most important message has been that schools *can* do this. And some of the schools that have made the greatest strides are the ones that are most resource-constrained."

Which is why, when asked about her hope for the program in the future, Lavizzo-Mourey can sum it up in one word: *sustainability*. "The schools that are adopting these changes ... have to figure out how it becomes just a part of the way they do their work, which is teaching kids. For us, it's spreading the idea widely enough that it can become the standard."

## Note

1. R. F. Wescott et al., "Industry Self-Regulation to Improve Student Health: Quantifying Changes in Beverage Shipments to Schools," *American Journal of Public Health* 102, no. 10 (October 2012): 1928–35.

# CHAPTER 9

# The Healthy Kids, Healthy Communities Program

*Marissa Miley*

## Introduction

In its efforts to improve the public's health, the Robert Wood Johnson Foundation has often looked to communities as proving grounds—places where different approaches could be tried, assessed, and, if appropriate, replicated.

When crack cocaine and other illegal drugs seemed to be tearing apart the nation's fabric in the late 1980s, the Foundation launched Fighting Back, a program that supported broad-based anti-drug and anti-alcohol coalitions comprised of local citizens, agencies, and organizations in fourteen communities.[1] Four years later, through a program called Free to Grow, it supported fifteen Head Start programs that organized coalitions of community leaders, social services agencies, and families to reduce substance abuse in their communities.[2]

In 1996, the Foundation launched the Urban Health Initiative, which engaged broad-based community coalitions in an attempt to measurably improve the health of children in five communities.[3] And in 1999, when the Foundation wanted to address pediatric asthma, it funded Allies Against Asthma; under the program, seven community coalitions developed ways to improve the environmental conditions that were known to trigger asthma.[4]

These are just a few examples of the Foundation's efforts to improve health by engaging community coalitions.[5] All told, the Foundation has spent well over three-quarters of a billion dollars supporting community coalitions.

In this chapter, Marissa Miley tells the story of the Healthy Kids, Healthy Communities Program, which ran from 2009 through 2014. Carried out in fifty communities (one dropped out before the program ended), Healthy Kids, Healthy Communities relied on broad coalitions of concerned citizens and organizations to improve the physical and social environment so that young people could get more physical activity and eat more nutritiously—and thus reduce childhood obesity.

Marissa Miley is an award-winning journalist specializing in science and health. Her honors include a 2014 GlobalPost Special Reports team award in public health reporting, presented by the Association of Health Care Journalists. She also co-authored the *New York Times* bestseller *Restless Virgins*. Miley was a Robert Wood Johnson Foundation Fellow at the Columbia University Graduate School of Journalism.

## Notes

1. I. M. Wielawski, "Fighting Back," in S. L. Isaacs and J. R. Knickman (eds), *To Improve Health and Health Care: The Robert Wood Johnson Foundation Anthology* Vol. VII (San Francisco: Jossey-Bass, 2004).
2. I. M. Wielawski, "Free to Grow," in S. L. Isaacs and J. R. Knickman (eds), *To Improve Health and Health Care: The Robert Wood Johnson Foundation Anthology* Vol. IX (San Francisco: Jossey-Bass, 2006).
3. P. S. Jellinek, "The Urban Health Initiative," in S. L. Isaacs and D. C. Colby (eds), *To Improve Health and Health Care: The Robert Wood Johnson Foundation Anthology* Vol. XI (San Francisco: Jossey-Bass, 2009).
4. A. Levy, "The Robert Wood Johnson Foundation's Efforts to Address Pediatric Asthma," in S. L. Isaacs and D. C. Colby (eds), *To Improve Health and Health Care: The Robert Wood Johnson Foundation Anthology* Vol. XII (San Francisco: Jossey-Bass, 2009).
5. For a discussion of community coalitions as a Foundation vehicle for improving health, see L. Leviton, "Engaging Community Coalitions," in S. L. Isaacs and D. C. Colby (eds.), *To Improve Health and Health Care: The Robert Wood Johnson Foundation Anthology* Vol. XII (San Francisco: Jossey-Bass, 2009).

J ust after seven o'clock on a mild October morning, April Robinson and her mother set out for the R. C. Hemphill Elementary School, a modest two-story brick building on a busy street in Birmingham's West End neighborhood. The nine-year-old April wears pink tennis shoes and a matching backpack, her hair neatly sectioned with plastic barrettes. Her mother, Olivia Boynik, dons an oversized T-shirt and red sweatpants. The logo emblazoned on her top ("If I'm Not Happy Nobody's Happy") belies her enthusiasm for the journey. "I know I don't have to do this," she says, "but it's something I like to do."

In a nearby parking lot, April and her mother greet several adults—some carrying small stop signs on wooden pegs, others wearing reflective fluorescent green vests—with the fluency of a three-year-old routine. As the sky brightens, they join the small volunteer crew of teachers, nonprofit workers, and at least one city official, and head down the street. Theirs has been the unofficial first stop on Hemphill's Walking School Bus, a once-a-week morning walk roughly two-thirds of a mile long. The Hemphill route, part of a national program encouraging walking or biking to school, was kick-started here across Jefferson County in 2011 with support from the Robert Wood Johnson Foundation.

As the group makes its way down Tuscaloosa Avenue to the public library, scores of children and a few parents, some arriving straight from night shifts, join the "bus." Their numbers swell with each bend in the road, a right on 14th Street and another on Fulton Avenue. Some children get out of cars pulled to the side of the road and others scramble down front porch steps. Adults and older children fan out to driveways and small alleys holding up the stop signs, and a lone policeman stands next to his car, the sedan's lights flashing silently.

The children's early morning conversations are bright and unencumbered, even as some of the sights they pass are not. April, her mother, and the nearly eighty other walkers pass some houses with caved-in roofs and others missing parts of their foundations. They step over scarred sidewalks and scattered piles of trash. In recent years, the West End has been synonymous with crime and general neglect. Around Hemphill, more than 40 percent of families with children under eighteen live below the poverty line, and nearly every student is eligible for the free school lunch program. Dozens of properties in the area surrounding Hemphill are tax-delinquent, resulting in blight that organizers say is unsafe for the children heading to school.

It is precisely this neighborhood's lack of so-called walkability that drew the Foundation to fund this initiative in the first place. The program under which the Walking School Bus took shape, called Healthy Kids, Healthy Communities, aims to help provide children like April Robinson with better options when it comes to their health. To those who have been walking along this route for the last three years, the options have visibly improved. A nearby community garden has supplanted an overgrown lot to become a neighborhood anchor, where a trained chef and self-professed "earth lover" introduces Hemphill students to vegetables like jicama and arugula. A row of orange traffic cones, new this year, lines the front of the school for children decamping the motorized school buses. The police officer, passive in the past, now scolds one father for permitting his kids to cross the street outside of the newly painted crosswalk.

Boynik wishes the Walking School Bus happened more than just once a week. She is concerned about her daughter's health. April has asthma, and despite the doctor's assurances, Boynik fears that the little girl, who is in the highest weight range for her height and age, is heading in the wrong direction. "I worry about her, period," she says. "That's my baby."

April appears to pay no mind, however. She scuttles ahead with a girlfriend to talk. It's the day before Halloween, and the fourth-grader has plans to be Hannah Montana. "I'm going to be a star," she says. Boynik, age fifty-three, trails behind, out of breath. The former city bus driver has type 2 diabetes and is on disability pay. But she does not complain. She has lost more than fifteen pounds in the last year. It all started with walking, she says, and modeling for her only daughter a life of activity and civic engagement. "It gets the adrenaline flowing, and it's good for my health to walk," Boynik says. "You have to show the children that it's all right."

## —∿— It Takes a Community

The Healthy Kids, Healthy Communities Program that galvanized the Walking School Bus and related activity in Birmingham and elsewhere across the country was a five-year, $33.4 million national initiative to promote healthy eating and physical activity changes at the community level.

The effort was shaped by past Foundation work tackling public health concerns like smoking and drug abuse, which had required decades of painstaking research and advocacy work in order to persuade policymakers to act. With childhood obesity, the Foundation sought to get to that policy action step faster. It wanted to fund something that would build a groundswell of momentum around childhood obesity prevention and would demonstrate what prevention strategies and tactics worked. The authority for change, the Foundation believed, was at the local level.

Beginning in the summer of 2008, the Foundation issued calls for proposals for the new Healthy Kids, Healthy Communities initiative. The term "community" was rather loosely defined; applicants were invited to submit proposals at the municipality, county, district, or regional level. They were encouraged to apply partnerships. The precise makeup of these partnerships was up to the community itself. What was nonnegotiable was that grantees would "implement healthy eating and active living strategies" that would build healthier communities. Toward that aim, they were to seek "integrated changes in policies, norms, practices, social supports, and the physical environment."

Initially, nine communities, from the Central Valley in California to Somerville, Massachusetts, were cherry-picked to apply as "leading sites." These communities, proven partners capable of spearheading and modeling work for others, would start a year in advance of the rest of the Healthy Kids, Healthy Communities grantees. When the program opened up to all communities across the country, 540 communities applied. But the Foundation could fund only a small number of them. The financial crisis had curtailed the program's reach, and ultimately, the Foundation funded, in addition to the nine leading sites, forty-one round-two sites.

The Healthy Kids, Healthy Communities grant ran from December 2009 through December 2013 (a supplemental grant running through the end of 2015 enabled the program to wind down in an orderly fashion). The national program office that managed the program, Active Living By Design, was located at the University of North Carolina's Gillings School of Global Public Health in Chapel Hill. The locale of the office was seemingly well suited for forging work in those Southern states where the childhood obesity epidemic was most pronounced. In its calls for proposals, the Foundation had sought grant applicants from particularly hard-hit states, including West Virginia, Kentucky, Mississippi, and Alabama.

The communities ultimately selected ranged from urban Philadelphia to rural Arkansas. The diversity was intentional. What the communities shared was their vulnerability to childhood obesity, whether by geographic location, poverty, race, or ethnicity. "These were not the low-hanging fruit," says Jamie Bussel, the Foundation's senior program officer for Healthy Kids, Healthy Communities.

Sarah Strunk, Active Living By Design's executive director, oversaw the fifty Healthy Kids, Healthy Communities grantees from Chapel Hill with just a handful of project officers, all of whom had backgrounds in public health or city planning. Active Living By Design specializes in the type of on-the-ground work that Bussel calls a "high-touch, low-dollar investment," characterized by providing frequent technical guidance and support to grantees. While the Healthy Kids, Healthy Communities program was one of the largest under the Foundation's childhood obesity commitment, it was distributed to grantees in relatively modest chunks over a period of four years. In total, each community received less than $400,000. "Anybody can do great things with millions of dollars," Strunk says. The challenge presented by the Healthy Kids, Healthy Communities grant was to ensure that efforts would continue long after the money dried up.

Whereas other significant national Foundation investments to reduce childhood obesity may have been narrowly focused in comparison, Healthy Kids, Healthy Communities was purposefully expansive. "We did not say, 'National program office, it's your job to reduce body mass index among children,'" says Dwayne Proctor, the Foundation's childhood obesity team director. "Their job was to make the opportunity available so that children could start to return to healthier weights."

And while the Foundation was not prescriptive in its specific tactics for prospective grantees, from the start it made clear that it wanted to create sustainable solutions, not one-off wins. Healthy Kids, Healthy Communities was not about getting a city to throw together an annual or even monthly running race, for example; it was about mobilizing community members to determine what kind of streets they wanted. Should there be more sidewalks? Less traffic? A crosswalk for children on their walk to school?

Grantees had to secure a matching cash or in-kind grant equal to at least 50 percent of the total Foundation grant, so it was critical for them to cultivate partners. The end result was collaborative but often messy, involving dozens of community partners and encompassing initiatives as diverse as working to change land use laws or encouraging local convenience store owners to stock their shelves with fresh produce. The work, too, was often incremental and the results fragile: community leaders come and go;

elected politicians turn over; promising youth advocates grow up and move away.

The idea behind the program was that even with these constraints, a critical mass of collective effort and policies will help reverse childhood obesity. "We really don't know what the mixture is in the secret sauce," says Risa Lavizzo-Mourey, president and CEO of the Robert Wood Johnson Foundation. "But we *can* say it's the comprehensiveness of the environmental change that seems to make a difference."

## —⌁— Jefferson County, Alabama

Jefferson County, Alabama, which encompasses the city of Birmingham, and, in turn, Olivia Boynik and her daughter, April Robinson's, West End neighborhood, was a round-two site. In 2009, when the Healthy Kids, Healthy Communities grant was awarded, Alabama was one of four states in the nation with obesity rates topping 30 percent; it also ranked number six on a list of states with the highest rates of overweight and obese children.[1] Not coincidentally, Alabama was among the states with the most diabetes, hypertension, and physical inactivity.

Jefferson County was emblematic of Alabama's entrenched problems. In its grant application, a young coalition of local foundations, government agencies, nonprofits, and grassroots organizations led by the United Way of Central Alabama and called the Health Action Partnership wrote that Jefferson County faced a number of barriers to healthy living, from unsafe parks to a lack of public transportation to a cultural preference for fried foods. There were other legacies to consider as well: in this county so deeply involved in the civil rights movement, impoverished neighborhoods like the West End have large concentrations of African Americans, and a mountain ridge geographically separates whites from blacks and the healthy from the unwell.

The Health Action Partnership saw Healthy Kids, Healthy Communities' focus on policy, systems, and environmental change as a critical way to "move long-term change," says Amanda Storey, who oversaw the first few years of the program in her capacity as assistant vice president of community health and wellness at United Way of Central Alabama.

As part, but certainly not all, of its plan to reduce and prevent childhood obesity, the Health Action Partnership aimed to make streets more walkable and bikeable and to connect the county's abundant parks and trails. Compared to forty years ago, when half of all children in the United States walked or biked to school, only 13 percent did so in 2009.[2] Alabama had been working to counteract this decline. Between 2005 and 2012, the state had received more than $17 million through the federal Safe Routes to School program that had allowed communities to pursue a host of changes, from repaving sidewalks to reducing traffic to creating routes that avoid abandoned houses. Those familiar with the Safe Routes program, however, found that resources were not being equitably allocated. "The money wasn't going to the areas where we felt the need was greatest," says Nick Sims, the Safe Routes coordinator for central Alabama.

With the Healthy Kids, Healthy Communities program, central Alabama had a chance to take advantage of the Safe Routes initiative. Like all grant applicants, the Health Action Partnership was required by the Foundation to complete a comprehensive assessment of its needs before embarking on any specific work. That rigorous process took a year, with partnership members reaching out to neighborhood associations, parent-teacher organizations, and after-school programs. What emerged was that residents of the West End and East Lake, the two communities core to the Healthy Kids, Healthy Communities grant, had expressed particular concern over school-related traffic and sidewalks. Back in 2007, a crossing guard at one school had even been hit by a car and killed.

Former director Amanda Storey first learned of the Walking School Bus at an annual Healthy Kids, Healthy Communities grantee meeting where the leading site, Columbia, Missouri, presented its work. Columbia had developed the "bus" with support from an earlier Active Living By Design grant, and had successfully leveraged that program to push through a $3.5 million sales tax to improve sidewalks around schools. Following that meeting, Storey returned to Birmingham energized. "This could be an answer to some of your needs," she recalls telling school officials. Soon members of the Jefferson County coalition began reaching out to the schools, including Hemphill Elementary School, proposing "Walking Wednesdays."

Janice Tyson, a Hemphill guidance counselor at the time, was at those early meetings. Known as a person who cares for the well-being of children beyond the boundaries of her job, Tyson was initially skeptical. "We had just had a terrible shooting in the neighborhood," she says. Four people had been hit, and one bullet casing had ended up in the school library. When the idea of "Walking Wednesdays" was presented, says Tyson, "We looked at each other and said, '*Walking?*'"

Still, sensing that this was an opportunity to do something new for the students, Tyson became a champion of the Walking School Bus. She brought then-school principal Gwendolyn Tilghman on board, and also asked several teachers to help out as volunteer chaperones. Parents, including Olivia Boynik, joined too. Bolstering the community involvement were volunteers from the Health Action Partnership, including from United Way, the YMCA, and the Jefferson County Department of Health.

The Hemphill Walking School Bus launched in the fall of 2011. Similar routes were initiated for two other schools. All routes were mapped to avoid dangerous areas, such as abandoned houses, and instead to pass by public buildings like the local library. When the children first started walking, they tiptoed around broken glass and walked past overrun lots. "It was awful back then," Tyson says. Storey recalls that only five kids showed up at first.

But over time, things started to improve. The commitment of community members has been particularly important. On a recent Wednesday, Alice Williams, a Safe Routes volunteer who also works in the mayor's office, was taking photographs with her smartphone of dead trees and piles of trash along the Hemphill route. Williams regularly e-mails pictures to city officials so that they can address such problems. Those might be safety hazards, cleanups, or properties to add to a list of condemned buildings. Even so, the challenge is enormous. "We've taken pictures ad nauseam," Williams says, estimating that some one thousand vacant properties remain on the city council's agenda.

The effectiveness of the Walking School Bus, as with Healthy Kids, Healthy Communities as a whole, relies upon the continued coordination of the community—from volunteers like Williams to committed parents like Boynik to the public works and public safety departments. Former Hemphill guidance counselor Tyson believes that this collective response—and the resulting improvements, from newly painted crosswalks to mowed vacant lots—ultimately helped the school stay open when a countywide bankruptcy forced others to close. Tyson, who now works at a different school, says that once the sidewalk is paved outside her new building, she hopes to launch the Walking School Bus there.

Having students walk en masse to school once a week may seem a quaint, even insignificant anti-obesity measure. The Healthy Kids, Healthy Communities coalition in Jefferson County started the Walking School Bus as a pilot program, and as of mid-2014, only four out of fifty-six schools in the district have implemented regular walks; three others have participated in a special "walk to school day." Getting parents to participate has been a constant struggle. Furthermore, studies have shown that the Walking School Bus alone is not likely to significantly increase physical activity or decrease obesity among children.[3]

In the city of Birmingham, however, the Walking School Bus is more than just a weekly walk—it's a community. Olivia Boynik feels so strongly about the program that she comes out every Wednesday, even though her daughter no longer goes to Hemphill. Beyond the walk itself, the program has had an impact. Former director Storey says that Jefferson County has been able to use the Walking School Bus to illustrate the need for "complete streets," or streets that take into account the needs of drivers, walkers, and everyone in between.

In 2012, Jefferson County was awarded $570,000 under the national transportation law that supported Safe Routes to School. The Healthy Kids, Healthy Communities initiative helped give teeth to a long-term city plan that would connect communities through walkable and bikeable paths across all twelve school districts in Jefferson County. The next step is to create a "safety zone" around schools like Hemphill, using a city ordinance that would expedite the cleanup of tax-delinquent properties, says United Way of Central Alabama's Kadie Whatley, who oversaw the grant program after Storey left.

A new federal transportation bill was signed into law in 2012, changing the grant structure for Safe Routes to School and its funding in Jefferson County. However, Safe Routes to School will be funded by a short-term grant through a different federal bill through March 2015. The Safe Routes to School program of Central Alabama is seeking new sources of funding to sustain its efforts and is housed by two partners in the Health Action Partnership: United Way of Central Alabama and the Regional Planning Commission of Greater Birmingham. Additional funding for related healthy initiatives has come from the Centers for Disease Control and Prevention (CDC) and the Community Foundation of Greater Birmingham.

## —∾— Charleston, West Virginia

Housed in an early-twentieth-century school building in a valley on the southwestern edge of West Virginia, the Mingo County Board of Education headquarters is so far off the grid that administrators have to trek miles into town to get the mail. The hour-and-a-half drive here from the state capital of Charleston takes you seventy miles down a stretch of highway where the only sights, apart from rolling mountains, are signs fast-food restaurants, and even they are few and far between. Then there's another fourteen miles on windy roads cutting through Appalachia, where logging and coal trucks seem bent on driving other vehicles off the road. There are no sidewalks in sight. The nearest grocery store is forty-five minutes away.

The surrounding rural area is best known these days for a political imbroglio; over the last year, murder, drug, and corruption charges among a handful of the county's elected officials have threatened to unravel this impoverished community of just twenty-six thousand on the border with Kentucky. The Mingo County Board of Education offices are, in other words, an unlikely setting for health innovation—as far-fetched a possibility, perhaps, as the name carved into the old building itself: Cinderella School.

But inside, on a recent Monday morning, more than three dozen teachers, principals, and wellness coaches nod in agreement as a petite Charleston pediatrician, Jamie Jeffrey, runs through a PowerPoint presentation she has put together on childhood obesity. Oversized portions of junk food, cuts to physical education and recess, and easily accessible sugar-sweetened drinks are all contributing to an "obesogenic environment," Jeffrey tells the group. "You can see why our kids are in trouble."

The Mingo County schools superintendent, Randy Keathley, asked Jeffrey to speak in her capacity as the project director for KEYS 4 HealthyKids, Charleston's Healthy Kids, Healthy Communities initiative. While West Virginia itself has among the worst figures for obesity in the nation—the highest rate of type 2 diabetes, the second-highest levels of physical inactivity, and the fourth-highest obesity rates in the country—the problems of Mingo County are particularly dire. Thirty-nine percent of its adults are obese and an equal percentage of fifth graders have high blood pressure. The county has among the lowest life expectancy rates for men in the United States—lower even than such developing world countries as Bangladesh.[4] In the face of these dismal prospects, Mingo County is trying to reverse poor health trends, and Superintendent Keathley hoped that Jeffrey could inspire and inform those educators in the audience.

Standing at the front of a large classroom, Jeffrey does not disappoint: she sports a chili-red blazer, orange moccasins, and bangs died pink for National Breast Cancer Awareness Month. In between sporadic "woo-hoos!" to commend Mingo County educators for their work so far, Jeffrey speaks as expertly about the biology of obesity as she does about the portion sizes at Olive Garden. If she had more than the two hours allotted, she likely would run through the two additional PowerPoint slide decks she brought with her on a thumb drive.

Though Jeffrey's energy level rivals the brightness of her outfit, she appears to connect most with the teachers when they lament the changes they have seen among their students of all ages. "The kids seem to be lazier," says one veteran physical education teacher. "It's hard to get them to be involved." "My kids groan when they have to get up to get a pencil," says another.

Jeffrey hears these complaints often, and knows well where the educators are coming from. She used to point fingers, too. A decade ago, as a pediatrician with the Charleston Area Medical Center, she began to notice a new normal among her patients. Most were trending overweight or obese. Increasingly, their measurements did not fit on standardized growth charts. They had adult health complications like high blood pressure and type 2 diabetes.

"I'm very much an authoritative pediatrician," Jeffrey says: "'This is what your problem is, this is what we're going to do about it, and this is what I need you to do.'" But telling her young patients and their families that they needed to lose weight just wasn't working. So Jeffrey dug into what little pediatric obesity science was available at the time, attended wide-ranging conferences long before there were specialized gatherings on the issue, and pored over medical studies and reports. Then she set up a multidisciplinary, yearlong weight-loss program that catered to kids and their families.

The initial outcomes were promising, but the long-term results were mixed; soon she saw that a costly "Cadillac program" wasn't going to address the childhood obesity problem on a broad scale. Most of Jeffrey's patients were from Charleston, many from the poor West Side. Ninety-three percent were on Medicaid. Overweight preschool-aged patients had little control over their diet or physical activity. Many well-meaning parents said they would buy more fruits and vegetables, but were unable to sustain it over time.

Something clicked with Jeffrey. Poor health "had more to do with the options in their communities than with their willpower," she says. That realization ultimately led her to team up with Judy Crabtree, head of the Kanawha Coalition for Community Health Improvement, a local community health group similar to Alabama's Jefferson County Health Action Partnership.

The Kanawha Coalition is an umbrella body of hospitals, schools, agencies, and charitable organizations. For the better part of a decade, it had identified obesity as the leading public health problem for Kanawha County, which encompasses Charleston. While the coalition had embarked on various short-term programmatic efforts around the issue, the Healthy Kids, Healthy Communities Program was an opportunity to create what director Crabtree calls "long-lasting changes."

On behalf of the new partnership between Jeffrey and Crabtree, the Charleston Area Medical Center Health Education and Research Institute, a nonprofit and educational arm of the hospital where both women worked, applied for the grant. Preparing the application alone took nine months and "a heck of a lot of partners, a whole lot of meetings, and a whole lot of late-night writing," says Jeffrey. As they wrote in their proposal, KEYS 4 HealthyKids would "unlock" the doors for "low-income kids and families to lead active, healthier lives."

The mnemonic KEYS reflected a program that was both kid-friendly and ambitious. The initiative would institute policy and environmental changes around "Knowledge," "Eating healthy," "Youth being active," and "Safety and empowerment." And it would start in three of the most impoverished neighborhoods of Charleston: the West Side, East End, and Kanawha City.

Like Birmingham, Charleston was a round-two site. Over the past four years, KEYS has benefited from the commitment of more than two dozen partners working across a range of health-promoting initiatives. They planted community gardens. They changed the nutritional makeup of handouts at a local food pantry. They developed a digital tool kit as a resource for other communities. Moreover, the KEYS program raised more than $300,000 in matching funds, along with some $200,000 in in-kind donations.

The work, while impressive, has not been without its headaches. "Any time you're working with communities," says Crabtree, "some folks are going to get it, others are going to take a while to get it, and others will never get it. You have to determine how to work with each of those populations to get to where you want to be."

Over the last several years, Jeffrey has become increasingly concerned about the prospects of younger children. Studies have shown that overweight or obese young children are five times as likely to become overweight or obese adults.[5] So Jeffrey has prioritized addressing obesity in children as young as two years old.

In Charleston's Kanawha City, in a tree-lined residential community on the south side of the Kanawha River, a class of preschoolers is finishing lunch at St. Agnes Child Development Center: a small cheese steak sandwich, baked wedge fries, a romaine salad, and an orange wedge along with 1 percent milk. The combination may not seem like the most virtuous of meals, but, says the day-care center's director, Sharon Bowles, for children who formerly were drinking sugary juice and eating iceberg lettuce and fried foods, these menu changes are substantial.

The more nutritious menu is just one of many changes that Bowles has made this year, following NAP SACC training that she and another teacher underwent with the KEYS team. The Nutrition and Physical Activity Self-Assessment for Child Care (NAP SACC) is a tool developed by researchers at the University of North Carolina at Chapel Hill, and is aimed at effecting lasting changes in nutrition and physical activity among young children. Heralded by First Lady Michelle Obama through her Let's Move! campaign, NAP SACC's principles were in line with those that Sharon Bowles had been trying to implement for four years, ever since she took the helm at St. Agnes daycare.

Jamie Jeffrey had first come across the NAP SACC program through an online forum and resource guide for Healthy Kids, Healthy Communities grantees. Deciding that this type of early childhood initiative would help create the foundation for a healthy life, in 2011 Jeffrey began conducting training sessions. At first they were one-on-one, but more recently she has staged group workshops over several days.

Throughout the NAP SACC assessment, which involves a comprehensive evaluation of food, screen time, playtime, written policies, and teachers' behaviors and knowledge, Bowles was appalled to learn how much of her kids' diet came from processed foods. She had thought that serving all-beef hot dogs was a good thing and that traditional West Virginia staples like biscuits didn't have much fat. She'd also believed that when the cook put French fries in the oven, that meant they were "baked." (In fact, they were pre-fried.) These revelations were particularly disturbing because most of the children under Bowles' watch are there for at least nine hours each day, eating the breakfast, lunch, and snack that the center provides.

In the school year that followed her NAP SACC training, Bowles guided St. Agnes to whole-grain breads and unsweetened cereals. The children now eat fresh produce three to four times a week, and they're no longer served their broccoli coated with cheese. During playtime, the children look forward to walks around the track with their teachers or to gymnasium sessions with hula hoops and jump ropes. The healthy changes that emerged from NAP SACC are visible within the classroom itself: in advance of the Halloween holiday, there is no candy to be seen. Instead, a crock-pot of homemade apple butter simmers on the counter to be canned and handed out to families, and a poster on the back wall features a dancing skeleton next to large cutout music notes and the words "Moving to the Beat!"

Undergoing NAP SACC training has had unanticipated effects outside of the day-care classroom as well: Bowles herself has lost twenty-six pounds, in part from abiding by the program's principles. A teacher who is overweight and diabetic told Bowles that the salad she gets at lunch is healthier than anything she could afford for herself at home. The children's parents have largely been supportive, says Bowles. It helps that she sends their kids home with monthly school menus, along with recipes for such healthy kid-friendly foods as Purple Cow fruit smoothies.

But for the St. Agnes child-care center to stay this more positive course, a champion like Bowles is crucial. These changes present challenges of their own, including the expense. Bowles says she spends at least an extra $100 a week on food, and now she has to pay the cook for an extra two hours a day to prepare the dishes. The changes are often time-consuming for her as well. The food vendor that serves St. Agnes doesn't always have the freshest, most affordable, or most appropriately portioned produce. As a result, Bowles spends an additional ten to fifteen hours a week of her own time hunting for recipes in cookbooks and online, scouring coupons, and running around to different supermarkets to take advantage of deals on healthy foods. At a recent excursion to her local Foodland, fresh pineapples were on sale for $2.99 each, cheaper than the canned version. "I just have to be on my toes and watch for things like that," Bowles says. On her desk, she keeps a thick stack of grocery store receipts. She puts in the extra time because "that's what the children need." But even with the center's largely middle-class families, says Bowles, parents will still pick up their kids and head to a drive-thru for dinner.

Continued improvement for St. Agnes is not guaranteed. While the day-care center was one of three schools in the past year to sign up for NAP SAAC training, Healthy Kids, Healthy Communities assistant project coordinator Laura Dice says the center has only recently completed the training and so far has changed only one written policy—one limiting sweets served during celebrations. Since St. Agnes is a parochial school, lasting change will depend on both the principal and the church finance committee continuing to approve the added costs. And, says Bowles, the cook will need to stay committed. "We'll be okay for at least the next year," she says. "And we'll just go from there."

So far, under Jamie Jeffrey's direction, eighteen child-care centers in the Charleston area have adopted NAP SACC. She hopes to convince the West Virginia Legislature to enact the child-care center initiative at the state level as well.

Meanwhile, far down in the southwest part of the state, Mingo County has absorbed the lessons from Kanawha County. And while Jeffrey's outreach to Mingo County doesn't fall under the Healthy Kids, Healthy Communities grant, it was informed and motivated by it. Mingo County school superintendent Randy Keathley says that Jeffrey's work through KEYS provides his school district with the evidence and know-how for implementing healthy eating and physical activity countywide. The county has already removed soda and sugar-sweetened beverages from its school vending machines, infused its school menu with whole-grain and lower-fat foods, and launched extended bus schedules so kids can participate in sports and play after school.

And Keathley says he'll continue working with Jeffrey to implement the KEYS policies even more fully. "Mingo County," Jeffrey says, "is one of the places that's doing it right."

## —⚏— Louisville, Kentucky

Michael Williams has just turned twenty-one. On a recent weekday he wears a button-down shirt and dress slacks, but in every other way he's the typical college sophomore: he likes to sleep until eleven o'clock on the mornings he doesn't have class; he squeezes in loads of laundry whenever he finds himself near his family home; and he wears his fraternity's letters—Phi Beta Sigma—prominently around his neck. And while he admits he's no health nut (he prefers fries to salad), Williams has been a leading advocate for changing the food options in his neighborhood of Shawnee, in the West End of Louisville, Kentucky.

By 2008, when Louisville was awarded a Foundation grant as a leading Healthy Kids, Healthy Communities site, the city already had a Foundation-supported Active Living By Design grant under its belt; that was awarded in 2003 for the purpose of improving the quality of the city's streets, enhancing its parks, and expanding fitness activities. And in 2004, Louisville saw the launch of the Mayor's Healthy Hometown Movement, a citywide effort that brought together diverse groups around a single goal: to make Louisville one of the healthiest cities in the country.

But, says LaQuandra Nesbitt, director of the Louisville Metro Department of Public Health and Wellness, that collective work often was "just a flurry of programmatic activity that needs to be funded year after year after year after year." The Foundation's Healthy Kids, Healthy Communities program enabled the city to think in a different, more collaborative and long-term way, Nesbitt says. Hers was the lead agency on the grant.

Louisville's new way of thinking also helped the city secure significant additional funding; from the CDC alone, Louisville received $7.9 million through the Communities Putting Prevention to Work Program and nearly $2.2 million through the Community Transformation Grant Program. Louisville was the only Healthy Kids, Healthy Communities leading site to be located in one of the fifteen states the Foundation had identified as bearing the brunt of the childhood obesity epidemic. Twelve neighborhoods, including Michael Williams' Shawnee, were the focus of the grant.

Several years ago, during the summer before his senior year of high school, Williams was looking to earn some extra money. In Shawnee, which has a majority African American population, more than a third of residents live below the poverty level. Only 9 percent of the residents have a Bachelor's degree or higher. Jobs are difficult to find.

Monica Brown, who runs the Shawnee Neighborhood Association, invited Williams to join a new initiative she was launching. At the time, her association had received funding from the Department of Justice as well as from the Center for Health Equity and the local YMCA, two partner organizations to the Healthy Kids, Healthy Communities Program. Brown saw that these grants could connect the dots between crime and health and provide much-needed employment for teenagers like Williams.

The neighborhood had been plagued by problems with drugs, gangs, and violent crime that made healthy living challenging, but the Shawnee Neighborhood Association had made headway by mobilizing to curb the sale of alcohol. That past neighborhood work enabled Healthy Kids, Healthy Communities to hit the ground running, particularly around healthy food access.

Both of Williams' parents had been professional cooks, but he had never seriously thought about the number of unhealthy chains and local fried chicken restaurants in his neighborhood. Louisville's ties to fast food run deep; it is home to YUM! Brands, owner of KFC, Taco Bell, and Pizza Hut. The local food store, Shawnee Market, was best known for selling beer and lottery tickets. It had never occurred to Williams that he was living in what public health professionals call a "food desert."

Beginning in 2009, during the summer and on weekends during the school year, Williams joined around twenty other teens in a community meeting space located in a strip mall. This was the Shawnee Neighborhood Association's headquarters, which doubles as a police substation. As part of their early work, Williams and his fellow teens went door to door asking residents what they wanted to see in their community. They documented with photos the physical contours of their neighborhood as well as the availability of food. They also participated in a walkability assessment, in which they noted the neighborhood's deteriorating sidewalks, missing curb ramps, and weedy areas, among other shortcomings.

At first, Brown says, the teens didn't understand how their work could possibly have an impact, but in time they grew to see the potential value of what they were doing. They ultimately named themselves the Shawnee Youth Advocates, and committed themselves to initiating change in their neighborhood around healthy food access, among other issues. Williams and his young colleagues created such momentum that they were even able to present the neighborhood walkability assessment to the Louisville mayor in a budget hearing.

An important activity for Williams involved improving the supply of healthy food at Shawnee Market, which, at the time, displayed bags upon bags of chips below a large sign advertising "Produce." Williams persuaded the store's owner, Akram Ali Al-Abed, to pilot a new program, "Healthy in a Hurry," to provide fresh produce for the neighborhood. With nearly $23,000 in funding through the Communities Putting Prevention to Work Program, Al-Abed bought refrigeration for fruit and vegetables.

Sasha Belenky, who worked on the initiative for the YMCA of Greater Louisville, helped Al-Abed make the space look brighter and more inviting: bottles of olive oil and seasonal decorations lined the top of the double fridge and nearby tables showcased potatoes and onions. For several months, Michael Williams worked in the store three to four days a week as the produce manager; he'd spent time at a local fruit and vegetable purveyor training for the job.

The outcome was so rewarding that Williams, Al-Abed, and the Shawnee Market were featured in a short documentary made by Active Living By Design. Williams was invited to speak at the Southern Obesity Summit, as well as at the annual Healthy Kids, Healthy Communities grantee meeting held in Louisville in May 2013. The work of the Shawnee Youth Advocates influenced other youth organizations, such as the new countywide Metro Youth Advocates run by the local YMCA with a grant from the US Conference of Mayors.

But the Shawnee Market has changed since the ending of the CDC funding and Healthy Kids, Healthy Communities Program, and that change illustrates the challenges for sustaining well-intentioned initiatives.

"At first everything was great," Williams says, listing the types of fresh produce available—oranges, grapes, squash, two different types of greens. "We'd get strawberries, and they'd be gone in two or three days." But walking through the dim, fluorescent-lit store for the first time in over a year, Williams can't hide his disappointment. He sighs at the sight of the half-empty refrigerator that contains only deeply bruised apples, wilted cabbage, and limp peppers.

The Shawnee Neighborhood Association's Monica Brown, who mentored Williams, believes that the store's "Healthy in a Hurry" sign—now prominently displayed next to advertisements for beer and meat—is a "false advertisement." Al-Abed, for his part, is let down, too. He says he gets produce shipments in once or twice a week, but "it's not moving well." He no longer buys items like eggplant or cauliflower without someone requesting them, because those items don't sell. When he buys a case of bananas, he can sell only half. The rest he throws away.

Al-Abed's store stands in sharp contrast to Webb's Market, a second-generation family-run store in the city's East End that also participated in "Healthy in a Hurry." Owner Tim Webb estimates that his business has increased some 30 percent through the "Healthy in a Hurry" initiative. In that case, the YMCA's Sasha

Belenky helped Webb reconsider his store design and layout, after which he moved the lottery machine to the middle of the store, removed bars from the windows, repainted the exterior, and took down the Budweiser sign out front. Now, despite his store's being only three thousand square feet, Webb estimates he sells up to $400 a week in produce.

Louisville's health director, LaQuandra Nesbitt, says that the mixed results of "Healthy in a Hurry" hold an important lesson for the city. "[Healthy Kids, Healthy Communities] was, I think, really a catalyst," she says, "because once you get out there and start knocking on doors and people say, 'I can't buy an apple,' you start trying to find solutions for it." The program helped Louisville draw funding from the CDC, which made working with store owners like Al-Abed and Webb possible. But for lasting change, Nesbitt says, there needs to be more than just money: "Here we had grant money, and we hung up a new shingle that said 'Healthy in a Hurry Corner Store.' We bought you a refrigeration unit, and we expected you to figure it out." These were stores that sold mostly packaged and canned food and whose owners were given little training to make fresh fruits and vegetables a cornerstone of their business.

The Shawnee Youth Advocates don't want to let up. Recently, they have expanded the scope of their work to other important issues, such as underage drinking and teen violence. But now they face an uncertain future, as funding has run out. Michael Williams still stays in touch, although his schedule at college keeps him busy. Working toward his degree in education, he has dreams of joining Teach for America. The former youth coordinator for the Shawnee Neighborhood Association, Kristen Lawrence-Williams, calls Williams an example of how young people can mobilize an entire community to act. "When kids notice, and take a stand," she says, "you have to answer that call."

## —ᨠ— Conclusion

The nine leading sites, including Louisville, largely wrapped up their work in 2012; funding for nearly all the remaining forty Healthy Kids, Healthy Communities grantees ended December 2013. Moving forward, the Robert Wood Johnson Foundation does not plan to expand to other communities using the same "high-touch, low-dollar" model. But it does seek to apply the program's lessons to its broader strategy of creating a national culture of health.

From the Foundation's perspective, the results from the program were positive. There were many "huge wins," says Jamie Bussel, the senior program officer who oversaw Healthy Kids, Healthy Communities. "It was a good program that worked," explains Foundation senior vice president Jim Marks. "But funding fifty more communities won't have the wide-ranging impact that is needed on thousands of communities." Thus, the Foundation, which recently completed a new strategic plan, is seeking to support communities in a different, more scalable way.

A St. Louis, Missouri-based consulting group, Transtria, is evaluating Healthy Kids, Healthy Communities, pulling data from the online dashboard that the communities used to connect with the national program office and other grantees and track their progress. Transtria is combing, coding, and assessing that data, but, says Allison Kemner, Transtria's project director for the Healthy Kids, Healthy Communities assessment, the idea is not to rank communities; it's to understand which changes and policies worked best in what setting.

While the firm's evaluation is still incomplete, it has counted more than twelve hundred policy and environmental changes, from creating community gardens (one of the most frequent changes) to improving corner stores and groceries (one of the least frequent changes). Although funding ended for one site because it was unable to carry on the work, the remaining forty-nine sites raised the requisite matching funding from local partners, even after launching during a deep recession. About a dozen communities received funding from the CDC's Communities Putting Prevention to Work program, and an equal number received CDC Community Transformation grants. Other communities have secured funding from entities outside of the health sector, such as the Department of Transportation. The many partnerships and coalitions formed, too numerous to count, brought into the fold for the first time nontraditional health allies like child-care centers, after-school programs, and parks and recreation departments.

In all of these measures of progress, however, one stands notably missing: documented changes in childhood obesity. But the Foundation, national program office, and grantees all say that measuring the prevalence of obesity with a hard number such as body mass index (BMI) was never the point. Nor was it even a useful measurement to consider for such a short-term grant. "The goal," says the Foundation's Marks, "was to change policies."

It is difficult, if not impossible, to tease apart the positive impact of Healthy Kids, Healthy Communities from the changed social and political landscape around childhood obesity in the United States. The five years of the program coincided not just with Let's Move!, but also with the White House Task Force on Childhood Obesity and the Partnership for a Healthier America, and with local initiatives throughout the country. Recent studies have found declining rates in childhood obesity, even, in some places, among those children most at risk.[6] "Attribution is always, quite frankly, very difficult," says the Foundation's Bussel. "Certainly contribution is a lot easier."

The communities themselves have, in many ways, spent the entire period of the grant preparing for the Foundation's departure. They know that the gains they achieved can be fragile, especially when there is no single project director or coordinator charged with rallying the troops. There is legitimate concern that even policies can be rolled back. But there is a stronger belief, and hope, that the policies and environmental changes will only move in a more positive direction. "With all of these funders and all of these initiatives, it's going to take time," says Jefferson County's Amanda Storey. "This is a complete culture change for all of us."

## Notes

1. J. Levi, et al., "F as in Fat: How Obesity Policies are Failing America," Trust for America's Health and the Robert Wood Johnson Foundation, July 2009, 10, 12.
2. http://www.saferoutespartnership.org/resourcecenter/quick-facts.
3. http://www.ncbi.nlm.nih.gov/pubmed/23079270.
4. http://www.pophealthmetrics.com/content/11/1/8.
   In 2010, men in Mingo County had a life expectancy of 67.26 years. H. Wang et al., "Left Behind: Widening Disparities for Males and Females in US County Life Expectancy, 1985–2010," Population Health Metrics, www.pophealthmetrics.com/content/11/1/8. Please see Additional file 1. Life expectancy for both sexes in every county across all years of the study (1985–2010). That same year, men in Bangladesh had a life expectancy of 69.5 years. World Bank, Life Expectancy at Birth, Bangladesh, http://data.worldbank.org/indicator/SP.DYN.LE00.IN/countries/BD-8S-XM?display=graph.
   Additional file 1. Life expectancy for both sexes in every county across all years of the study (1985–2010). Men in Mingo County had a life expectancy of 67.26 in 2010. Also in 2010, men in Bangladesh had a life expectancy of 69.5.
   http://data.worldbank.org/indicator/SP.DYN.LE00.IN/countries/BD-8S-XM?display=graph
5. R. C. Whitaker, et al., "Predicting Obesity in Young Adulthood from Childhood and Parental Obesity," *New England Journal of Medicine* 337 (1997): 869–73. As referenced by the Centers for Disease Control, http://www.cdc.gov/mmwr/preview/mmwrhtml/mm6231a4.htm?s_cid=mm6231a4_w.
6. Centers for Disease Control, "Vital signs: obesity among low-income, preschool-aged children, 2008–2011," *Morbidity and Mortality Weekly Report*, August 9, 2013, http://www.cdc.gov/mmwr/preview/mmwrhtml/mm6231a4.htm?s_cid=mm6231a4_w.

# Section Three
# Local Initiatives

# The 211 LA Developmental Screening and Care Coordination Program

*Digby Diehl*

## Introduction

Nearly thirty years ago, the Robert Wood Johnson Foundation first funded the Local Initiative Funding Partners Program. This unique effort—in which the Foundation shared the funding of promising community programs with state and local foundations—enabled the Foundation to reach deep into communities and nurture ideas that germinated locally.[1]

The Local Initiative Funding Partners Program and its successor, the Robert Wood Johnson Foundation Local Funding Partnerships Program, generated many remarkable programs and inspiring leaders, some of whom have been featured in the *Robert Wood Johnson Foundation Anthology*. These include Jim Kinyon, whose Catholic Social Services brought mental health and substance abuse counseling to the Lakota Sioux living on or near reservations in South Dakota;[2] nurse practitioner Martha Ryan, who started San Francisco's only prenatal care clinic for homeless women and saw it mushroom into a $1.7 million operation with thirty employees serving eighteen hundred homeless families;[3] and pediatrician Darcy Lowell, whose Child First program to prevent mental health problems in high-risk children proved so effective in Bridgeport, Connecticut, that it was expanded throughout the state and beyond.[4] These are just a few examples of the kinds of leaders and projects that the Local Initiative Funding Partners Program and the Local Funding Partnerships Program looked for and supported.

In this volume, we are highlighting a Local Funding Partnerships Program effort called the 211 LA County Developmental Screening and Care Coordination Program. Under the dynamic leadership of Maribel Marin, one of its founders, and Patricia Herrera, its director, the program has transformed a traditional telephone helpline ("211") into a screening and referral service for young children with autism and other developmental disabilities. Since its beginning in September 2009, the program has screened nearly eight thousand children under the age of five; nearly half of them were found to be at moderate to high risk of a development delay.

Digby Diehl wrote the chapter on the 211 LA County Developmental Screening and Care Coordination Program in this volume. A frequent contributor to the *Anthology* series, Diehl has collaborated on many books, including *Rather Outspoken* (with Dan Rather); *The Million Dollar Mermaid* (with Esther Williams); and *Angel on My Shoulder* (with Natalie Cole). His most recent collaboration is *Alone Together: My Life with J. Paul Getty* (with Theodora Getty Gaston). It was published in 2013 by HarperCollins.

## Notes

1. I. M. Wielawski, "The Local Initiative Funding Partners Program," in S. L. Isaacs and J. R. Knickman (eds.), *To Improve Health and Health Care: The Robert Wood Johnson Foundation Anthology*, Vol. III (San Francisco: Jossey-Bass, 2000).
2. D. Diehl, "The Catholic Social Services Outreach Project," in S. L. Isaacs and D. C. Colby (eds.), *To Improve Health and Health Care: The Robert Wood Johnson Foundation Anthology,* Vol. XII (San Francisco: Jossey-Bass, 2009).
3. D. Diehl, "The Homeless Prenatal Program," in S. L. Isaacs and J. R. Knickman (eds.), *To Improve Health and Health Care: The Robert Wood Johnson Foundation Anthology,* Vol. VII (San Francisco: Jossey-Bass, 2004).
4. D. Diehl, "Child FIRST: A Program to Help Very Young At-Risk Children," in S. L. Isaacs and D. C. Colby (eds.), *To Improve Health and Health Care: The Robert Wood Johnson Foundation Anthology*, Vol. XV (San Francisco: Jossey-Bass, 2013).

"My name is Latonia Jenkins. I have two sons. The oldest, DeMarcus, is three-and-a-half, almost four years old. His brother Amare is eighteen months. Amare is fine, but I called 211 LA because I have some concerns about DeMarcus. He has a very limited vocabulary. He points to things he wants, rather than saying what they are. He says "123 ABC," but not too much more than that, and he keeps repeating the same things over and over. He doesn't know how old he is, he can't tie his shoes, and we're still working on potty training."[1]

Roughly one out of six children in the United States has autism, cerebral palsy, a learning disorder, or another developmental disability, but these problems are not evenly distributed throughout the population.[2] They are also not evenly diagnosed. Children from low-income families, particularly ethnic minority children, are doubly vulnerable. Not only are they at greater risk for developmental disabilities, they are also less likely to have their problems addressed in a timely manner.

More than 115,000 of these at-risk children live in the County of Los Angeles. To help identify them and connect them with services, a pediatric developmental screening program was launched in 2009. What makes this program unique is that screenings are not conducted face-to-face in clinics or doctors' offices, but over the phone by 211 LA County (211 LA), an information and referral call center. Officially known as the Developmental Screening and Care Coordination Program, it is the first and thus far the only such program in the nation. Robert Wood Johnson Foundation funding for the program began in 2010 and concluded in 2013.

Patricia Herrera has administered the program since its inception. Fluently bilingual, with graduate degrees in both counseling and psychology, she is an advocate for her program and for the families it serves. "I know it can be a challenge for parents to get help for children with a developmental delay or disability," she says. "There is always a lot of bureaucracy and red tape to deal with. Having worked in this field for years, it has been my experience that, generally, the parents who are best able to get services are the ones with the most resources. Their English is good. They know how to work the phones; they know how to fill out paperwork. They don't take 'no' for an answer.

"In contrast, many of the neediest families in Los Angeles County do not have these skills or resources. It's hard, sometimes impossible, for them to get connected with agencies that can help them—those who are most in need are also the most likely to get shut out. These are the families who call 211 LA every day. We have to make the system more equitable, so that the haves and the have-nots are both getting services at the same rate. This program is a step toward that goal."

A private, not-for-profit 501(c)(3) organization serving the ten-plus-million residents of the Los Angeles metropolitan area, 211 LA fields half a million calls a year. Callers reach out to 211 LA for assistance in dealing with a broad spectrum of life issues, from landlord disputes and problems with disconnected utilities to substance abuse and domestic violence. Operating around the clock seven days a week, it is staffed by approximately seventy specially trained operators called Information and Referral (I & R) Specialists. They listen to callers describe their situations and then refer them to the appropriate agencies for assistance. Specialists are bilingual (English and Spanish), but information can be conveyed in any of about 140 languages through an on-call interpreting service. The 211 LA call center also serves the hearing impaired.

The center began in Los Angeles in 1981 with support from United Way, and was initially called Info Line. Maribel Marin became executive director in 2002. With a Master's degree in urban planning and extensive work experience in public works and contract administration, she brought a canny business sensibility to the delivery of social services. Early in her tenure, she moved to replace the jumbled collection of toll-free 800 numbers with the all-inclusive 211 designation. "Two-one-one is so easy to remember," says Marin. "As soon as we converted, we started to be inundated with calls. We doubled our size, and doubled our budget." With the transition, the service changed its name to 211 LA and joined a fledgling nationwide network of 211 call centers. That network has since expanded to cover more than 90 percent of the US population.

To solidify the financial stability of 211 LA, Marin negotiated sole-source contracts with a variety of government agencies. Funding for the call center is now assured by multi-year agreements with various Los Angeles County agencies, including the Department of Mental Health and the Department of Children and Family Services. In addition, 211 LA is written in as an integral component of the county disaster response network, providing an information resource in the event of an earthquake, wildfire, or other emergency. Marin was able to leverage that designation to procure a generator, paid for by the US Department of Homeland Security, to power 211 LA headquarters, which is located in what was formerly a savings and loan. "Because we are part of disaster response, we need an independent source of electricity," she says. "Even if the power goes out—especially if the power goes out—we must be able to keep functioning."

To offer callers concrete, specific support in time of need, I & R specialists tap into a catalogue of available services. In Los Angeles County, that includes nearly fifty thousand programs administered by five thousand federal, state, and local agencies. In an effort born of necessity, Marin directed her staff to create a comprehensive electronic database of these services to help I & R specialists cut through the tangled web of overlapping programs and jurisdictions.

Called the "Taxonomy of Human Services," this database functions much like a card catalogue in a library. Just as the nationwide Dewey Decimal System guides readers to the books they want, whether they are searching the vast holdings of the New York Public Library or the stacks at the local community college, the taxonomy gives I & R specialists detailed descriptions of agencies and programs. It is continually reviewed and revised as government programs and eligibility criteria evolve. Maintaining its completeness and accuracy is now a full-time job for five 211 LA staff resource writers.

Because of its consistent, comprehensive listings and descriptions, the taxonomy has been adopted as the national standard by the Alliance of Information and Referral Systems, the accrediting body of 211 call centers. All certified I & R specialists across the country are versed in how to use it. This common organizational framework and common descriptive language enables I & R specialists to pitch in during emergencies taking place hundreds or thousands of miles away. This is an essential capability in times of disaster, when local 211 centers can be either swamped by the volume of calls or out of service entirely. When Hurricanes Gustav and Ike hit Louisiana in 2008, calls to overwhelmed 211s along the Gulf Coast were rerouted to 211 LA, together with their local database of services.

## —∿— Bringing Developmental Screening to 211 LA

Implementation of the pediatric developmental screening program has its roots in the Los Angeles Early Identification and Intervention Collaborative (the collaborative). The collaborative began in the fall of 2003 with a group of ten health and social welfare professionals brainstorming over lunch about how to identify children with developmental delays at an earlier age. Since that first luncheon gathering, the collaborative has grown to become a loose coalition of more than 350 agencies and service providers, including education, public health, and law enforcement, all of whom are affected by the problem.

Jeanne Smart, a registered nurse who heads the Los Angeles County Department of Public Health Nurse-Family Partnership Program, is a longtime collaborative member and former committee chair. "The collaborative came together when it was becoming obvious in every system of care—public health, mental health, school systems, foster care—that there were so many children who were not developmentally appropriate," she recalls. "All of us were seeing children who were severely developmentally delayed—not rolling over at an appropriate age, not sitting up. Most of them had never been tested, not even the ones who had received some kind of regular pediatric attention. Doctors simply were not doing developmental assessments. They were telling parents of preschoolers—kids who weren't talking, not even babbling—that their children were going to be 'fine.' This didn't happen just once or twice; it was chronic. And it is still common today."

Frustrated by the systemic failure to identify these children, members of the collaborative started exploring alternatives to clinic-based assessment. "The prospect of developmental screening outside the clinic or doctor's office presented a chance to make a difference," says Smart, "but the idea of putting it in 211's lap came from Margaret Dunkle."

As the catalyst behind the formation of the collaborative and its founding director, Margaret Dunkle had a particular interest in finding a new mechanism to reach underserved communities. "In 2003, we in the collaborative started thinking about policies and strategies that would help us find these children," she recalls, "but it took more than five years of groundwork to get the effort launched. Developmental screening can be done effectively in a lot of settings. One place where it *should* be done is during a child's regular pediatric visit, but we know it's not being done there."

Olga Solomon, a University of Southern California researcher specializing in autism, echoes this assessment. "In Los Angeles and across the country, children with developmental disabilities are not getting identified soon enough to benefit from early intervention," she says. "Even when parents notice the first signs of autism and point them out to their pediatricians, it's all too common for doctors to discount or dismiss their concerns."

Some of this may be attributable to the fact that pediatricians, like many physicians, are overscheduled. "In this era of the fifteen-minute doctor visit," continues Solomon, "pediatricians complain that they don't have enough time. And many of them are not well enough connected to resources in the community to know where to refer children who need help, even if they do identify them."

Although a 211 call center had never been used for pediatric screening, there was a compelling demographic argument in favor of trying to make it work. Out of the half million calls 211 LA fields annually, about 85 percent are from women. More than three-quarters of all callers are Latino or African American. Most are low or very low income—55 percent of them are trying to get by on less than $1,000 a month. More than eighty-four thousand calls per year come from parents with children under the age of five. In short, 211 LA serves the neediest families in the county—the families that are both at greatest risk and least likely to have access to pediatric developmental screening.

The involvement of 211 LA in developmental screening dates from June 2006, when Maribel Marin first attended a meeting of the collaborative. "While we were in the process of converting our phones, transitioning out of the old 800 numbers and into the 211 role, we began to do outreach to inform all of our partners that this was happening," she says. "At about the same time, the collaborative was going through its strategic planning process. The collaborative approached us because they thought we might be able to help them identify children with developmental delays. We sensed an opportunity. We knew from our caller surveys that we were reaching a large number of lower income families with children under five. We knew that these were families with high psychosocial risk factors. We didn't know how to do developmental screening for young children—yet—but we knew that we had the families that everybody was looking for."

"This," says Margaret Dunkle, "was when things started to come together. The following year, federal legislation was amended to require high quality developmental screening in all Head Start programs. Finally there would be a real obligation to address the need that we in the collaborative had seen for so many years."

At Dunkle's suggestion, 211 LA asked Patricia Herrera, long a collaborative participant, to head the program. Herrera came to 211 LA from the Frank D. Lanterman Regional Center, one of twenty-one regional centers in California. Regional centers are private, nonprofit corporations that are run under the auspices of the State Department of Developmental Services; they work with individuals who have lifelong developmental disabilities.

Herrera initially joined the 211 LA developmental screening program as a consultant; her first responsibility was to find a way to fund it. With assistance from Dunkle, she began writing grant applications. In December 2008, the W. M. Keck Foundation awarded 211 LA a start-up grant of $300,000. "We knew that children were not getting screened until they were in kindergarten or first grade," says Dorothy Fleisher, program director for Keck's Early Learning Program. "By that time, they were already years behind. Beyond the importance of the program, however, we were very impressed with the dynamic leadership of 211 LA."

With initial funding assured, Herrera was officially named director of the Developmental Screening and Care Coordination Program. The Weingart Foundation provided a one-year grant of $106,000 in June of 2009. "This was an opportunity to support an area of work that the Weingart Foundation has long been interested in," says Belen Vargas, the foundation's vice president of programs. "It was a chance to really address some of the issues concerning how and why it has been difficult to get young children screened. There are so many lost years during which intervention services could have changed their story."

The Robert Wood Johnson Foundation became involved in 2010, when its Local Funding Partnerships Program awarded the program a three-year grant of $500,000. (The Keck Foundation served as the program's nominating funding partner.) "We wanted to test the model to see whether people would call in to 211, and to see whether families would be able to get screened and then be connected with service providers," says Pauline Seitz, director of Local Funding Partnerships. "Our goal was to learn whether this was a model that would work in a community as large and complex as greater Los Angeles."

## —∞— Early Intervention—the Stitch in Time

Why are early identification and early intervention so important? Biomedical research has proven that by the age of three, 80 percent of human brain development is complete. The very young brain adapts and responds to new stimuli, which makes the ages from birth to five, and in particular the ages from birth to three, the prime time to help a child who is exhibiting signs of developmental delay or autism. The window of opportunity starts to close thereafter, limiting not only the chances of success, but also the amount of improvement that can be achieved. "The benefits of early identification and early intervention are huge," says Charles Sophy, Medical Director for the County of Los Angeles Department of Children and Family Services. "The first five years are the key time frame to lay the foundation for all of the stuff that goes into making a solid human being—trust, integrity, self esteem. The younger the age, the more positive impact intervention will have."

"Early intervention," says Margaret Dunkle, "is often the critical stitch in time that can make a huge difference in a child's development." Autistic children in particular benefit greatly from intensive early intervention. Recent research shows that not only can it improve their language and social skills, it can also actually normalize brain activity.[3] As autism researcher Olga Solomon says, "It literally may make the difference between a child who grows up to assemble and pack boxes in a sheltered workshop, and a child who goes to college."

# —ᴍ— Developmental Screening

Developmental screening at 211 LA begins with what might be considered a typical 211 call.

> "You've reached 211 LA. This is Linda. How can I help you today?"
>
> "My name is Yolanda Zamora. I need to find housing right away for me and my son."
>
> "I can assist you with that, Ms. Zamora. What is your current situation?"
>
> "I'm in a shelter. I left home because my husband is doing drugs. He's been getting into fights, even when Javier, our son, was watching. I didn't feel safe anymore."

The first priority of the I & R specialist is to take care of the original stated reason for the call. Beyond responding to the original request, the specialists are trained to probe for unstated needs. Callers asking about food assistance may also get information on how to file for Medicare or Medi-Cal, or for veteran's benefits, or how to get immunizations or a flu shot. And even when the caller doesn't volunteer the information, all I & R specialists routinely ask whether there are children under the age of five in the home. "People who are struggling often do not have a real understanding of what services are available," says Herrera. "We give them as many resources as we can, and while we're at it, we ask them about their kids. That's what makes the developmental screening model so powerful, because it flows from their own original request."

So after Linda helped Ms. Zamora get connected with resources for permanent low-income housing, she gently asked about her son:

> "While I have you on the line, Ms. Zamora, may I ask whether you have any concerns about how your son is developing?"

"Yes I do, actually. It's very hard to understand what Javi is saying. I've already brought it up with his pediatrician, but the doctor said she didn't see anything wrong."

Linda then offered Ms. Zamora the opportunity of getting a developmental screening for Javier, eventually patching her through to one of 211 LA's care coordinators.

I & R specialists do not follow a script, but there are protocols in place for dealing with each type of call the center receives. This includes a standard procedure for handing off a caller to a care coordinator for developmental screening, making a "warm transfer" whenever possible. If a care coordinator is available, the specialist makes the introduction and passes the caller on; the interaction briefly becomes a three-way conference call:

> "This is 211 LA County. My name is Cheryl. How can I help you today?"
>
> "My name is Graciela Flores. I need help getting back-to-school supplies for my child."
>
> "I'd be happy to assist you with that, Ms. Flores. May I have your zip code, please?"
>
> "91106."
>
> "That's Pasadena. I can give you a list of places where you will be able get backpacks, notebooks, and other supplies. Will your child also be needing immunizations?"
>
> "Yes."
>
> "Okay, Ms. Flores, I will also be giving you a list of clinics where you can get the immunizations that your child will need for school. While I have you on the line, Ms. Flores, do you have any concerns about how your child is developing?"
>
> "I do, actually. Miguel is four years old and he's not talking in complete sentences."

"Ms. Flores, 211 Los Angeles County offers developmental screening for children under the age of five. If you are interested in that screening, I can connect you with one of our care coordinators."

"I am interested, yes."

"Ms. Flores, I'm going to put you on hold briefly while I contact one of our care coordinators. Please stay on the line . . . . Ms. Flores, I have Nancy, one of our care coordinators, here. She will help you with the developmental screening. Nancy, this is Graciela Flores. Her son Miguel is four years old."

"Good afternoon, Ms. Flores. My name is Nancy. I understand that you are concerned that your son may have speech problems . . . ."

As the developmental screening program was gearing up, the team had to decide what screening methodology would be used. Margaret Dunkle believed that a parent questionnaire developed by Frances Glascoe, a professor of pediatrics at Vanderbilt University, could be adapted for use by 211 LA. Called PEDS (Parents' Evaluation of Developmental Status), the screening test consists of a series of standardized questions designed to elicit parents' concerns about how their child is progressing.

The PEDS test has two critical assets: brevity and accuracy. Just ten questions long, it detects 70 to 80 percent of a wide range of developmental and behavioral issues. Although PEDS had already been rigorously tested and validated, it had never been administered by phone before. Its use by 211 LA would break new ground.

Glascoe consulted with 211 LA on the use of her model throughout the first three years of the program. She believes that phone screenings actually offer some distinct advantages. "When doing the assessment over the phone, the care coordinator can encourage the parent to give a lot of information. We've found that parents are eager to talk about their children. If a mother says that her son is three years old and hyperactive and doesn't sit still for a minute, the care coordinator will take note of that, even if the parent says she is not concerned about it."

Care coordinators, all of whom are bilingual, must have a college degree in early childhood education or in some aspect of social work, psychology, or family therapy. They must be familiar with risk conditions for developmental disabilities, and must have some direct counseling experience. It is also essential that they possess excellent listening skills and a great deal of empathy; they need to be able to make parents feel comfortable talking about their children, particularly if the parent suspects there may be a problem.

Care coordinators are trained to project a phone personality that is warm and conversational—professional, but never clinical or judgmental. Nancy Godoy, who helped Ms. Flores in the situation above, began her career in case management at Harbor Regional Center and has been a care coordinator with the 211 LA developmental screening program since it began. "We make sure that the caller feels heard, and that we are addressing what he or she believes is a concern. Many parents who call us, particularly younger parents, do not have a good grasp of what constitutes age-appropriate development. For this reason, speech and communication problems are often the first issue to get their attention."

As the screening proceeds, care coordinators continually feed the parents' responses back to them: "*Okay, Ms. Flores, what I hear you saying is*...." This gives the parent the opportunity to correct or clarify any misunderstanding, and also to add additional information. "At first I was very surprised by how much parents would tell me over the phone," says care coordinator Irene Aceves. "People share things about their household, their family, the way they are living their lives. Mostly, though, they like talking about their kids."

What do care coordinators listen for? "There are things a parent might say that would raise a flag," says Nancy Godoy. "When a mother says, 'He's in his own world,' I will ask whether she can tell me more. If she says, 'I can't handle him anymore. He's out of control,' I might say, 'Let's talk about the behaviors. What is he doing exactly? How often is he doing it? Is it just with you, or is it at school?' Sometimes it's the parent who needs some parenting skills. Other times, there really is something going on with the child, and the child needs intervention, or the child has a condition that needs to be diagnosed."

Care coordinators also have to "listen between the lines," says Godoy. "We can't focus solely on a child's speech difficulty, even if this is the parent's primary reason for calling. Being behind in language development could be a speech problem in and of itself, but it could also be an indicator of other issues. We need to understand why the child is behind. We have to take into account everything that's going on in the child's life."

## —∿— Neither Diagnosis Nor Prescription

As soon as the screening is completed, care coordinators share and discuss the results with the parent. Following their established protocol, they speak to the child's strengths first, before addressing the problems. Coordinators then work with the parent to develop a plan of action. "We work it out so that there is a consensus between the family and the coordinator," says Patricia Herrera, "with the coordinator using her best informed judgment about what will work for the family."

Herrera is careful to point out that screening and referral constitute neither a diagnosis nor a prescription. "From that perspective, 211 LA has always been protected from liability," she says. "We are simply providing parents with options, and informing them about how to pursue them. We say that if the screening finds something, there's reason for you to be concerned, and doctors and clinicians should take a closer look at your child."

Care coordinators are always mindful that the results of the screening may be difficult for a parent to hear and accept. "There's a denial that's to be expected," says Irene Aceves. "Veronica was a parent I screened almost a year ago. I referred her to a Head

Start Early Education program, to her local school district, and to a regional center, because there were a lot of concerns. She followed through just with the Head Start, but actually that was great, because once you get into Head Start, they also do a screening. The staff there started telling her that her son needed further testing. Just last week she called me back. 'You know what, I'm embarrassed,' she said. 'I'm ready for the referral to the regional center now.'"

For Latonia Jenkins, the mother at the beginning of this chapter, the results were surely not what she was hoping to hear. Although she suspected that DeMarcus, her older son, had developmental problems, she didn't initially have concerns for her younger son, Amare. But after Amare's screening, she learned that he had failed the autism screening test. Faced with two children with developmental disabilities, Latonia decided to "think a little" about whether to accept the referral to a regional center.

Patricia Herrera nevertheless remains hopeful for the family. Like Veronica, Latonia Jenkins was connected to a Head Start, where both of her children will receive assessments. "Our goal is not to get everyone to a regional center," says Herrera. "Our goal is to get these children the services they need."

Care coordinators offer resources to parents even when the screening does not indicate a significant risk of developmental delay. Paula Dinkins, a student, called 211 LA because she was looking for low-income housing for her family and for child care for her two young children. After the I & R specialist provided her with that information, Dinkins accepted the chance to do a developmental screening with Irene Aceves. She admitted that she was somewhat concerned because Curtis, her two-year-old son, was throwing tantrums and displaying aggressive behavior.

Although neither Curtis nor Emily, his older sister, was found to be at risk for developmental delay, Dinkins did eventually reveal what might be part of the problem: she and her children were living with her parents, who had stopped admitting Dinkins' day-care provider into their home. This was why she was looking for low-income housing. "I have night classes," she says. "I often don't get home till 11:00 p.m. I just want my kids to sleep in their own beds at night." Irene Aceves was able to connect Dinkins with parenting classes to help her cope with Curtis's tantrums and aggression.

## —∿— Care Coordination—Active, Hands-On Referral

Once the screening is completed, care coordinators need to deploy an additional set of crucial skills. "Our care coordinators must understand how social services are delivered," says Maribel Marin, "and in Los Angeles County, that can be very complicated. To be able to help someone over the phone, you have to know how to work the system."

In the words of the 211 LA Web site, care coordinators "locate, refer, broker, monitor, expedite, provide advocacy, and coordinate fragmented services offered by professionals and organizations from different disciplines. They also provide information and coaching to parents and caregivers on navigating the service system."

Political geography, combined with the situations of the callers, can make the care coordinator's task more difficult. Los Angeles County is a crazy quilt of jurisdictions with irregular boundaries, including incorporated cities, unincorporated areas under direct county governance, and school districts. Who is responsible for delivery of services to an at-risk child is often dependent on the family's place of residence, but many callers to 211 LA don't have a permanent address. Often it's part of the reason they're calling; they could be staying in a motel or a shelter, or couch surfing, or they may be living in their car.

Moving frequently and not having proof of residence can be a serious barrier to receiving services, and it is a problem that care coordinators frequently have to overcome. Learning how to connect at-risk children to resources effectively takes specialized study.

"Our care coordinators go through a rigorous five-week training program before they get on the phones," says Marin, "but training doesn't ever really stop. We have anywhere from two to ten hours a month of follow-on training to keep everyone on top of what's happening."

One of the much-praised facets of the 211 LA developmental screening program is the hands-on connection of families with service providers. Care coordinators direct their families not just to an agency, but to a particular person in the agency. Whenever possible, they are on the line with the parent when that connection is made. The process is in many ways parallel to the warm transfer between the I & R specialist and the care coordinator that precedes the developmental screening.

"With referrals from clinics and physicians, there is a general tendency not to follow through," says Vanderbilt's Frances Glascoe. "Often they don't make the recommendation strongly enough, or they just hand families a phone number. That just never works. What 211 LA does is stay on the phone with the family when they make a referral. They link them live to Head Start, to Early Start, to regional centers. Their uptake is more than twice that of primary care providers."

"Here at 211 LA," says Patricia Herrera, "we know that if you tell a mother her child may have a developmental problem, you better know where to send her. We not only give her a referral, we'll tell her who she's supposed to see, what papers she'll need to bring, the hours the office is open, and what buses she'll have to take to get there. If she needs a bus fare, we'll tell her how to get it. That's what care coordination is."

And it doesn't stop once the referral has been made. Coordinators stay in touch with the family, not just to make sure that the referral handoff has been successful, but also to buttress the health and stability of the family as a whole. On average, care coordinators make seven follow-up calls with the families they have screened. "We stay in contact," says care coordinator Godoy, "Until we know they are receiving some kind of intervention services—preschool, mental health, speech therapy, assessment at the regional center. We also invite them to call us. We are working in partnership to help their child."

## —∿— A Performance-Driven Organization

The 211 LA developmental screening program sprang from the cooperative efforts of the many agencies participating in the Early Identification and Intervention Collaborative. Once the program was launched, Marin and Herrera built on that legacy of teamwork, working with and through the collaborative to establish a strong network of partnerships with service providers.

The program has cemented those partnerships with memorandums of understanding (MOUs). Although nonbinding, the MOUs codify how the agencies work together. Partner agencies commit to taking 211 LA referrals and providing outcome information, and 211 LA commits to doing the screening and to providing care coordination and a care plan for the family. Partner agreements are in place with all seven regional centers in Los Angeles County, with the Los Angeles County Office of Education, and with a number of Head Start and Early Head Start providers. More are pending.

The MOUs are "the acknowledgment that we both have the same mission: to find these children and serve them," says Herrera. "We have real relationships with our partners—we did a lot of meaningful work together before we had the piece of paper."

Much of this "meaningful work" involved laying the groundwork for a relationship of trust. Before committing to take referrals from 211 LA, receiving agencies had to have confidence not just in the integrity of the screening process, but also in the ability of care coordinators to make sure that the families they refer are qualified to receive services. "Assessment and early intervention can be costly," says Marin. "A comprehensive assessment at a regional center involves a physician, a clinical psychologist, and a speech therapist. The cost averages $8,000 per child. With that kind of expenditure, our partners need to know that we aren't sending them families who don't match their eligibility criteria."

211 LA's extensive data collection and analysis system helps to reassure its partners. From the outset, 211 LA has made data a priority. "We are a performance-driven organization, so we know that operations need to be driven by outcomes—and for that you need data." For the developmental screening program, 211 LA developed its own software to track information about parents participating in the program, as well as about care coordination. New information is automatically integrated into 211's existing electronic database, allowing 211 LA to follow the children it refers to the partner.

## —⚬— The Road Ahead

After nearly a decade of screening and making referrals, those responsible for LA 211 have gained many insights. "I think the first lesson we learned," says Herrera, "and it was a big question at the outset, is that families, even in their most stressful situations, still want to talk about their children. The tool that we use allows us to have those conversations in a very compassionate, caring way, so that families feel connected to us, and are willing to take the next step."

The second lesson came from an unforeseen statistic. Approximately 70 percent of the parents who accepted the offer of developmental screening didn't initially make contact because they were concerned about their child's pace of development. Most, like Yolanda Zamora looking for housing or Graciela Flores in search of school supplies, called for other basic needs.

Above all, the 211 LA developmental screening program confirmed the great number of children in need of early screening and intervention. The results from the first four years of the program—from September 2009 through June 2013—are striking. Of the 7,816 children whose parents completed the screening, more than half were found to be at moderate to high risk for developmental delay or disability, and almost a quarter were identified as being at high risk. This is roughly twice the rate found in the population as a whole. And of the more than 4,800 children screened for autism, 16 percent were found to be at high risk, a rate one and a half times greater than the national rate. For most of these families whose children were identified as being at risk, the findings were completely unexpected—only about a third of parents who participated had expressed concerns about their child's development before the screening took place.

211 LA would like to expand, but does not yet have the budget to offer screening to all parents of young children who call in. "We get seven thousand callers with children under five each month," says Patricia Herrera. "At present we are screening between 10 and 12 percent of them. It's a drop in the bucket, but our capacity is limited because at present we can only carry three care coordinators on staff." The philanthropies that originally backed the 211 LA developmental screening program are no longer funding it. Financial support for the program now comes primarily from a grant from First 5 LA, a county commission that is funded by California's tax on tobacco products. Although support from First 5 will sustain the screening program at its current level for the near future, Marin and Herrera are exploring a number of alternatives that would eventually give the program greater financial independence.

The first is by forging partnerships with universities and other research institutions. Academic researchers know that good data are hard to come by. For them, the trove of information 211 LA receives from its high volume of callers, coupled with its built-in system for electronic collection and analysis, is a mother lode. For 211 LA, published research papers based on its aggregated data are expected to offer a real opportunity to enhance the credibility and reputation of the developmental screening and care coordination program. "Our university partners have seen the potential for this to be a best practice," says Herrera. "It's a win-win."

The program is now expanding its partner relationships to include universities and research institutions. In 2013, it began a new partnership with the UCLA Kaiser Permanente Center for Health Equity. The first step is a study conducted by Bergen Nelson, an assistant clinical professor of pediatrics at UCLA and former Robert Wood Johnson Foundation Clinical Scholar, that will utilize 211 LA's data to evaluate the effectiveness of the developmental screening and care coordination program. "We understand the value of performance- and evidence-based practices," says Marin. "Within 211 LA, we already have great confidence in the effectiveness of our model, but there is a difference in perception between our saying what our data show and UCLA independently confirming what our data show. We anticipate that their rigorous analysis will validate our model. At that point, we will be in a stronger position to increase our screening capacity and attract more government support."

In addition to the relationship with UCLA, 211 LA has established similar data-sharing agreements with several of its community partners, including the LA County Office of Education, Head Start, and all seven regional centers in the county. The organization is in discussion with several other institutions, including the University of Southern California and Children's Hospital Los Angeles. Other cities have also approached 211 LA about replicating the program outside California. There have been exploratory discussions with cities in Pennsylvania, Michigan, and Missouri.

One of the first efforts at replicating the developmental screening model may take place within 211 LA itself—but with a different target population. Marin is looking to adapt the pediatric developmental screening model to other populations, including veterans and, through Head Start, homeless families who have children in need of early intervention. "After homeless shelters make a referral, care coordinators will do the screening," says Los Angeles County Head Start Director Keesha Wood. "They will automatically refer them to Head Start. We will start working with them, and then give that information back to 211. It's a program that has great potential. If we can make it work successfully here in LA, which is huge, we can be a model for other communities."

A key objective in securing the future of the 211 LA developmental screening program is to tap into reimbursement funding based on federal and state mandates. "We're trying to focus on the programs that are already allocating money for the activities that we think we can do better," says Herrera. As part of its partnership with UCLA Kaiser Permanente, 211 LA is looking to undertake care coordination for several of its pediatric community clinics. "We know that pediatricians do not have the infrastructure to organize screening for low-income families, nor do they have the ability to offer care coordination," says Marin. "We already have a system in place that is efficient and consistent—and we can track data." Because these clinics are publicly funded, 211 LA would be positioned to receive reimbursement under both Medi-Cal and the Affordable Care Act. The Individuals with Disabilities Education Act (IDEA) offers another possible revenue stream. The law stipulates that children with disabilities are entitled to early intervention and special services that are designed to prepare them for further education. Each state is charged with implementing a comprehensive, coordinated effort to provide services. Through a provision called Child Find, school districts are required to be active in identifying all children who need early intervention. In California, the state's program to address their Child Find obligation is called Early Start. "It is a funded mandate," says Herrera, "but there has been a lack of coordination among agencies receiving Child Find monies. Bureaucracies tend to work in isolation, in silos. It's very inefficient, both in terms of identifying children and in terms of best use of resources."

## —∿— Conclusion

There is broad consensus among child development experts that pediatric screening should be universal for all children. "The earlier the identification, the earlier the intervention, the better the outcome," says Maura Gibney, family resource manager of the South Central Los Angeles Regional Center. "With the right early intervention by occupational therapists and physical therapists, we can often make up the delay. We can set these children on the road to a full and productive life."

"The greatest potential for 211 LA lies in its ability as a single organization to marry screenings with referrals to services," says Paul Chung, associate professor of pediatrics and chief of general pediatrics at the David Geffen School of Medicine and Mattel Children's Hospital at UCLA. "Screening is worthless unless you can get people connected to services, and getting people connected to services is worthless unless we can figure out who needs to get connected. That's the magic that 211 has the potential to deliver. For a large number of families who have been left out of access to these services, 211 might turn out to be their best bet."

The implications of revamping the approach go far beyond developmental screening. With the adaptation of the model to use with veterans and with homeless families, the 211 LA developmental screening program suggests a new, more efficient, more effective way to integrate service providers and find economies of scale in the process. As 211 LA says on its Web site, they are looking toward "changing the system, one child at a time."

## Notes

1. Latonia Jenkins is a pseudonym, as are the names of other callers in the chapter.
2. C. A. Boyle, et al., "Trends in the Prevalence of Developmental Disabilities in US Children, 1997–2008," *Pediatrics* 127, no. 6 (2011): 1034-42.
3. http://www.ucdmc.ucdavis.edu/publish/news/newsroom/7079.

# —ww— The Editors

*David C. Colby*, PhD, a distinguished health care expert who joined the Robert Wood Johnson Foundation in 1998, is its first-ever vice president of policy. Working between Washington, D.C., and the Foundation's headquarters in Princeton, New Jersey, Colby oversees what he describes as a "two-way street" sharing of information and expertise between the Foundation and Washington policymakers, interest group leaders, and others. In his tenure at the Foundation he has held a number of leadership positions, most recently the vice president of research and evaluation. He came to the Foundation after nine years of service with the Medicare Payment Advisory Commission and the Physician Payment Review Commission, where he was deputy director. Earlier he taught at the University of Maryland, Baltimore County, Williams College, and State University College at Buffalo. Colby's published research focused on Medicaid and Medicare, use of emergency departments, AIDS, and various topics in political science. He was an associate editor of the *Journal of Health Politics, Policy and Law* from 1995 to 2002. He received his doctorate in political science from the University of Illinois, a Master of Arts from Ohio University, and a Bachelor of Arts from Ohio Wesleyan University.

*Stephen L. Isaacs*, JD, is a founding partner of Isaacs/Jellinek, a San Francisco-based consulting firm that works with foundations and not-for-profit organizations, and president of Health Policy Associates, Inc. A former professor of public health at Columbia

University, he has written extensively for professional and popular audiences. His book *The Consumer's Legal Guide to Today's Health Care* was reviewed as "the single best guide to the health care system in print today." His articles have been syndicated and have appeared in law reviews and health policy journals. A graduate of Brown University and Columbia Law School, Isaacs served as vice president of the International Planned Parenthood Federation's Western Hemisphere Regional Office, practiced health law, and spent four years in Thailand as a program officer with the US Agency for International Development.

# —᠊ᨠ— The Contributors

*Joe Alper* has been a science writer and technology analyst for over thirty years. He played a central role in planning and establishing the National Cancer Institute's Alliance for Nanotechnology in Cancer and Physical Sciences-Oncology Centers programs, as well as the National Institute of Mental Health's Decade of the Brain initiative, and has written numerous policy documents for the President's Council of Advisors on Science and Technology (PCAST), the National Cancer Institute, the National Institutes of Health, and the National Academies of Science, as well as many other foundations and federal agencies. He has also served as a contributing correspondent for *Science* and as a contributing editor of *Nature Biotechnology* and *Self* magazines, and has written for a variety of publications, including *the Atlantic Monthly*, *Harper's*, the *New York Times*, the *Washington Post*, and *Nature Biotechnology*. He graduated from the University of Illinois at Urbana-Champaign with a BS in chemistry, and received MS degrees in both biochemistry and agricultural journalism from the University of Wisconsin-Madison.

*Will Bunch* is senior writer for the *Philadelphia Daily News* and has won a number of national and regional journalism awards, including sharing the 1992 Pulitzer Prize for spot news reporting while at *New York Newsday*. He has written for a number of top publications including the *New York Times Magazine*, the *Washington Post*, *Mother Jones*, the *American Prospect*, and Salon.com, and is a front-page blogger for the Huffington Post. He is the author of a popular blog, *Attytood*; three books, including *Tear Down This Myth: The Right-Wing Distortion of the Reagan Legacy* and *The Backlash: Right-Wing Radicals, High-Def Hucksters, and Paranoid Politics in the Age of Obama*, on the rise of the Tea Party; and two Amazon Kindle Singles.

*Digby Diehl* is a writer, literary collaborator, and television, print, and Internet journalist. His book credits include *Rather Outspoken*, the *New York Times*–bestselling memoir of journalist Dan Rather; *Patti LuPone: A Memoir*, written in collaboration with one of Broadway's foremost leading ladies; *Priceless Memories*, the autobiography of Bob Barker; *Remembering Grace*, a look back at the life of Grace Kelly (with Kay Diehl); *Angel on My Shoulder*, the autobiography of singer Natalie Cole; *The Million Dollar Mermaid*, the autobiography of MGM star Esther Williams; *Tales from the Crypt*, the history of the popular comic book, movie, and television series; and *A Spy for All Seasons*, the autobiography of former CIA officer Duane Clarridge. For eleven years, Diehl was the literary correspondent for ABC-TV's *Good Morning America*, and was the book editor for the *Home Page* show on MSNBC. Previously the entertainment editor for KCBS television in Los Angeles, he was a writer for the Emmys and for the soap opera *Santa Barbara*, book editor of the *Los Angeles Herald-Examiner*, editor in chief of art book publisher Harry N. Abrams, and the founding book editor of the *Los Angeles Times Book Review*. Diehl holds an MA in theatre from UCLA and a BA in American Studies from Rutgers University, where he was a Henry Rutgers Scholar.

*Paul Jablow* is a freelance journalist who spent more than three decades as a newspaper reporter and editor with the *Charlotte Observer*, the *Baltimore Sun*, and the *Philadelphia Inquirer*. Since leaving the *Inquirer* in 2003, he has been a consultant writer for the Robert Wood Johnson Foundation, an investigator for the Philadelphia Board of Ethics, and, most recently, a member of a research team at the Children's Hospital of Philadelphia working on a federally funded project to bridge the linguistic gap between clinicians and patients. He lives in Bryn Mawr, Pennsylvania.

*Risa Lavizzo-Mourey* is president and CEO of the Robert Wood Johnson Foundation, a position she has held since 2003. The Robert Wood Johnson Foundation is the nation's largest philanthropy dedicated solely to health and health care. With more than thirty years of personal experience as a medical practitioner, policymaker, professor, and nonprofit executive, Lavizzo-Mourey has built on the Foundation's forty-year history of addressing key public health issues.

A specialist in geriatrics, Lavizzo-Mourey came to the Foundation from the University of Pennsylvania, where she served as the Sylvan Eisman Professor of Medicine and Health Care Systems. After attending the University of Washington and the State University of New York at Stony Brook, Lavizzo-Mourey earned her medical degree from Harvard Medical School. She also holds an MBA from the Wharton School at the University of Pennsylvania. Lavizzo-Mourey is a member of the American Academy of Arts and Sciences; the Institute of Medicine; the President's Council for Fitness, Sports and Nutrition; the Smithsonian Institution Board of Regents; and several boards of directors.

*Marissa Miley* is a Boston-based journalist and deputy editor of global health for special reports at *GlobalPost*. Her reporting honors include a team award in public health reporting from the Association of Health Care Journalists. She also coauthored the *New York Times* bestseller *Restless Virgins*. Miley has received journalism fellowships from the United Nations Foundation (2013), the Kaiser Family Foundation (2013), and the International Reporting Project (2014), through which she has reported untold public health stories on the ground from Zambia to Brazil and in the United States as well. She is a graduate of the Columbia Graduate School of Journalism, where she was a Robert Wood Johnson Foundation Fellow in science and health writing.

*Tony Proscio* is a senior fellow at the Center for Strategic Philanthropy and Civil Society at Duke University's Sanford School of Public Policy and a consultant to foundations and major nonprofit organizations. He offers strategic consulting on program design, planning, and evaluation; communication; and policy analysis and development. He is coauthor, with Paul S. Grogan, of the book *Comeback Cities: A Blueprint for Urban Neighborhood Revival,* and has written three essays on civic and philanthropic jargon published by the Edna McConnell Clark Foundation. Previously, he was associate editor of the *Miami Herald,* where he was lead editorial writer on economic issues and wrote a weekly opinion column.

*Sara Solovitch* is a writer whose stories have appeared in *Esquire, Wired, Outside,* and other publications. She has been a staff reporter at several newspapers, including the *Philadelphia Inquirer,* and has had numerous stories published in the *Washington Post* and the *Los Angeles Times.* For six years, she wrote a weekly column on kids' health for the *San José Mercury News.* She has just completed her first book, an exploration and memoir of stage fright, which will be brought out by Bloomsbury Publishing in June 2015.

*Irene M. Wielawski* is an independent writer and editor specializing in health care and policy topics. She has written extensively on socioeconomic issues in American medicine, particularly the difficulties faced by people without timely access to medical services because of financial, geographic, cultural, and other barriers. Wielawski was a staff writer for nearly twenty years for daily newspapers, including the *Los Angeles Times,* where she was a member of the investigations team. Subsequently, with a research grant from the Robert Wood Johnson Foundation, she tracked local efforts to care for the medically uninsured. Other commissioned projects include producing pediatric medicine segments for public television, an analysis of the Massachusetts health reform law, and collaboration on the redesign of the classic business school case study for use in graduate-level health professional studies. Her independent work appears in the *New York Times*, the *Los Angeles Times*, and *Kaiser Health News*, among daily outlets, on Web sites, and in peer-reviewed journals and books. Wielawski has been a finalist for the Pulitzer Prize for medical reporting and shared in two *Los Angeles Times* staff Pulitzers, among other honors. She is a founder and current board member of the Association of Health Care Journalists, a reviewer for *Health Affairs*, and a graduate of Vassar College.

*Amy Woodrum* is currently a program associate at the Robert Wood Johnson Foundation. She works with colleagues in the executive office, helping to implement Foundation and program strategy. Since joining the Foundation, she has helped connect lessons from across its areas of focus and understand how the Foundation can improve its grantmaking practices.

Prior to joining the Foundation, Woodrum graduated from the University of Pennsylvania with a BA in Health and Societies. She spent time working at the Center for High Impact Philanthropy in the University of Pennsylvania's School of Social Policy & Practice, and as a social performance intern for Kiva, a microfinance organization in San Francisco. Woodrum also received a certificate in Core Public Health Concepts from the University of North Carolina, Chapel Hill.

# —∿—Index